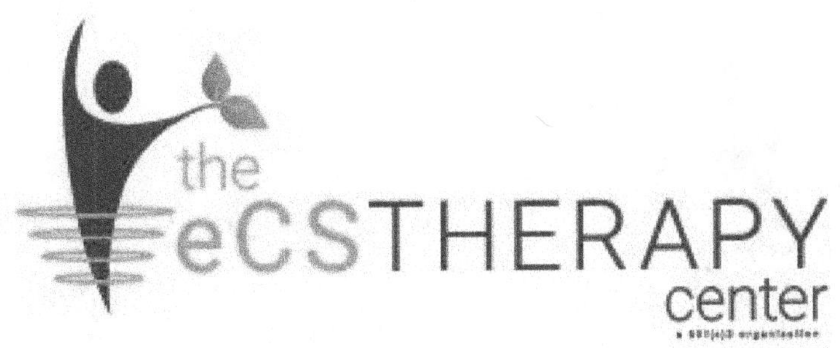
the
eCSTHERAPY
center
a 501(c)3 organization

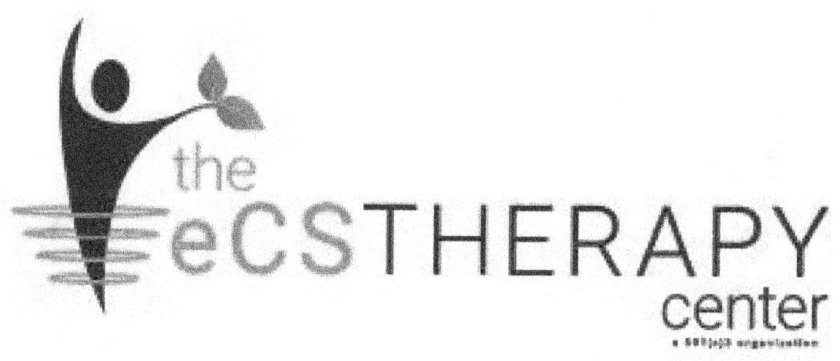
the eCSTHERAPY center
a 501(c)3 organization

BY: DR. REGINA NELSON

CANNACIAN® LEVEL ONE HANDBOOK

Offered by The eCS Therapy Center

WWW.MYECSTHERAPY.ORG

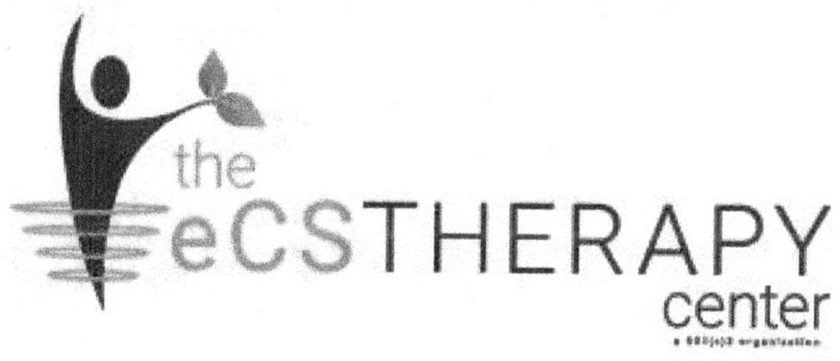

Cannacian® Certification
offered by
The eCS Therapy Center and
Certified Cannacian® Trainers

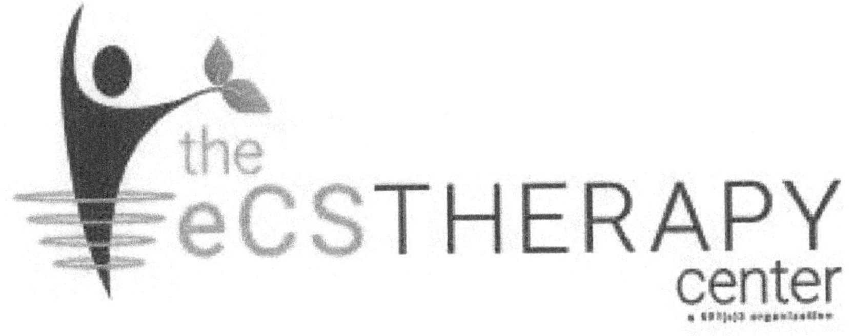

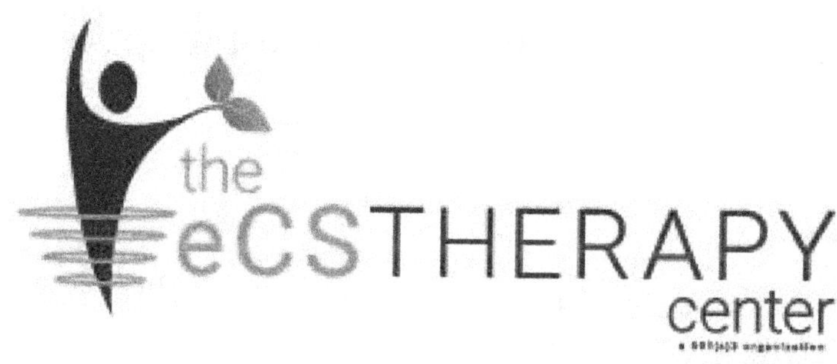

Cannacian® Level One Certification

Author: Regina Nelson, Ph.D.
President, The eCS Therapy Center

ISBN: 9798831977547

The Cannacian® Level One Training is offered
by The eCS Therapy Center, Dr. Regina Nelson, and certified
Cannacian® Trainers.

Each section of courses has been accredited for Continuing
Medical Education (C.M.E. - American Academy of Family
Physicians) and Continuing Education (C.E. by multiple
accrediting agencies). Due to the accreditation
the Cannacian® program is offered to the public as a
certification by The eCS Therapy Center (a national 501c3
organization).

All curriculum has been written by Dr. Regina Nelson. Dr.
Nelson is not a medical professional but has earned a Ph.D.
in Ethical and Creative Leadership. She is an educational
leader in the cannabis industry and a medical cannabis
patient.

Originally Published August 2019, Updated 2022

WHAT IS A CANNACIAN®?

A COACH OR COUNSELOR EDUCATED AND KNOWLEDGEABLE ABOUT THE USE OF CANNABIS AS MEDICINE.

CANNACIAN® CERTIFICATION OFFERED BY THE ECS THERAPY CENTER AND FROM LICENSED CANNACIAN® TRAINERS WORLDWIDE.

WWW.MYECSTHERAPY.ORG

Cannacian® Level One Certification

- Time for the Talk: Doctor-Patient Communication
- An Introduction to the eCS
- Hemp v. Cannabis: What's the difference?
- Targeted Dosing Strategies

Cannacian® Level Two Certification

- An In-Depth Look at the eCS
- Cannabis Therapy Planning
- Pediatric Cannabis Use
- Veterinary Cannabis Use

Cannacian® Level Three Certification

- Cancer & Cannabis
- Cannabis Therapy Planning for the Chronically Ill
- Opiate Withdrawal & Dependence and Cannabis
- Seniors and Cannabis

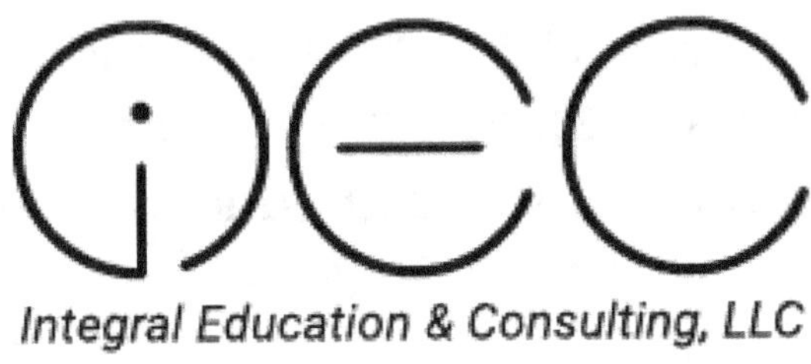

Integral Education & Consulting, LLC

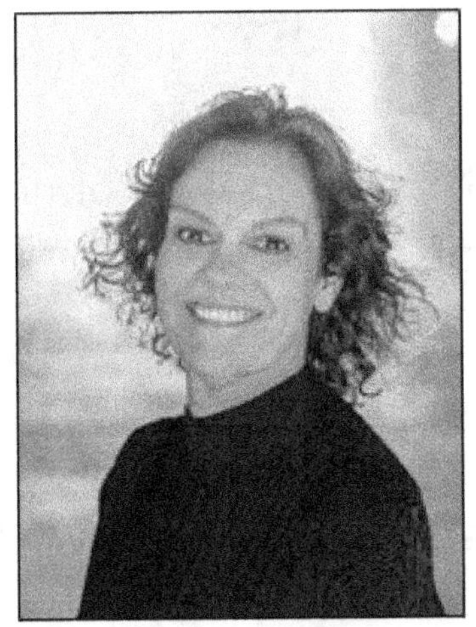

DR. REGINA NELSON earned her Ph.D. in Ethical and Creative Leadership at Union Institute and University in 2016. Her doctoral studies concentrated on Medical Cannabis. She has been publishing peer-reviewed articles since 2012, engaged in national cannabis education since 2013, and began presenting topical research projects in 2015. Nelson is a well-recognized public speaker in leadership, public policy, Integral theory, public health, and cannabis arenas.

Dr. Nelson founded The eCS Therapy Center in 2015 and currently sits as the President of the Board of Directors. She is also the author of multiple titles including: *Theorist-at-Large: One Woman's Ambiguous Journey into Medical Cannabis, The Medical Cannabis Recommendation: An Integral Exploration of Doctor-Patient Experiences*, and *The Survivor's Guide to Medical Cannabis*.

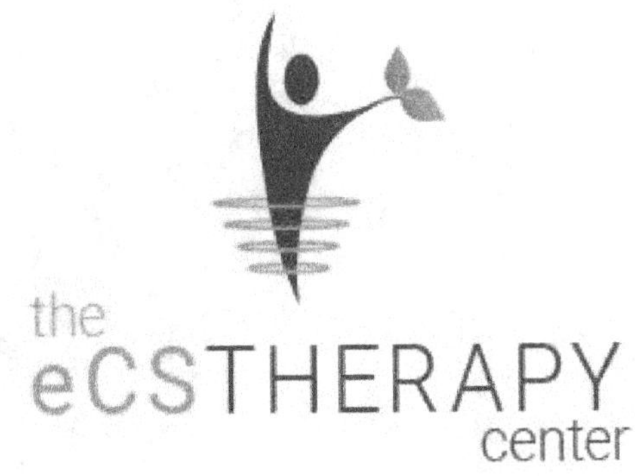

Dr. Nelson is a Founding Officer and current President
of The eCS Therapy Center a 501(c)(3) Integral organization
- national champion of community-based education and
research projects.

www.myecstherapy.org

She also leads Integral Education & Consulting, LLC as C.E.O.
providing cannabis consulting services, private education
for organizational groups, and leading research projects for
cannabis organizations.

www.IntegralEducationandConsulting.com

Much of the information regarding the endocannabinoid
system (eCS) or the use of cannabis as medicine are
referenced from Dr. Nelson's book, *The Survivor's Guide to
Medical Cannabis*.

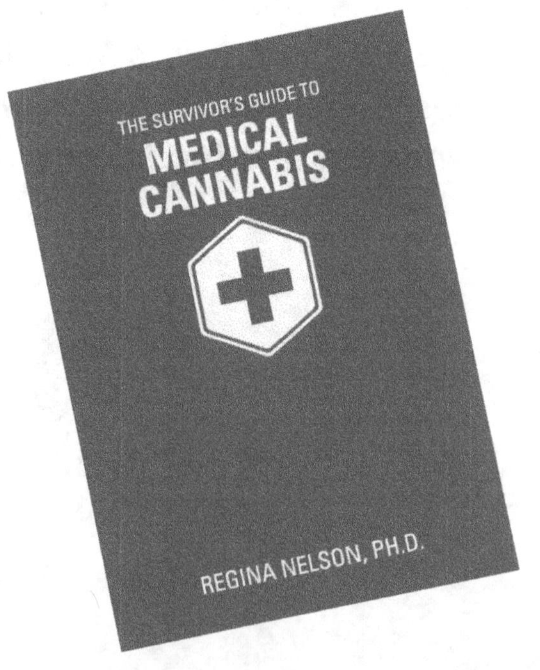

**2nd Edition
Due Summer 2022**

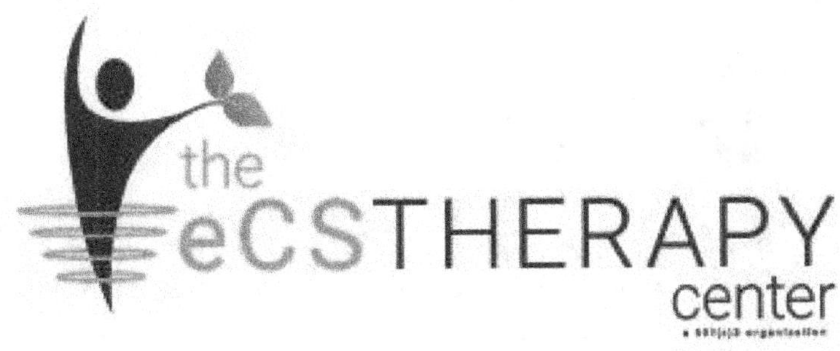

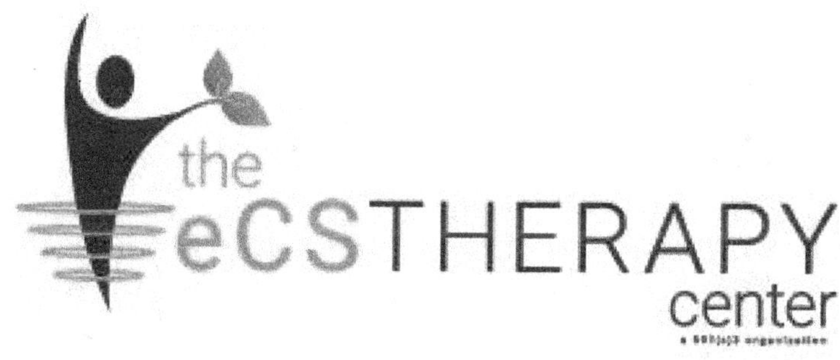
the
eCSTHERAPY
center
a 501(c)3 organization

Welcome to
Time for the Talk: Communicating with Your Doctor or Patient about Medical Cannabis

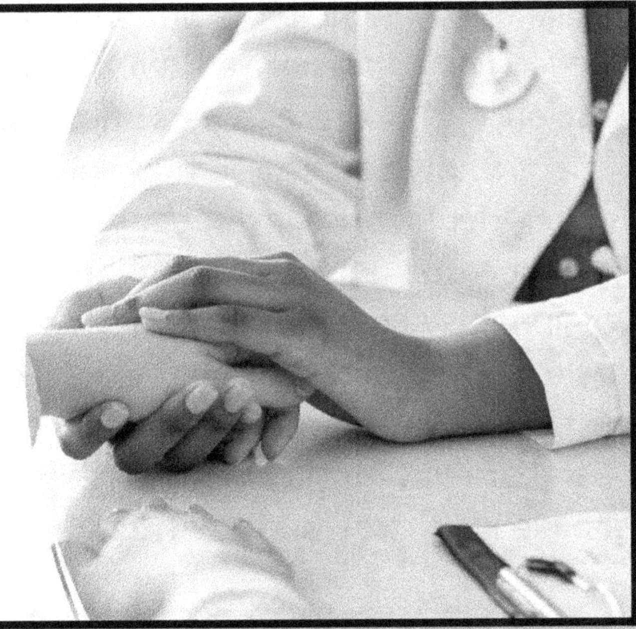

Personal Introduction by Dr. Regina Nelson

I always like to begin with a disclaimer: I am not a medical doctor, but that I am a Ph.D. in Ethical and Creative Leadership and a medical cannabis patient.

I began my journey into medical cannabis in 2010. Though I had been a long-time cannabis user, I'd become sick and I was looking for answers. Because I could find so little research, especially social research on the subject, I chose it as the topic to focus my degree in Ethics & Social Justice.

As a desperate patient in search of answers, I began attending the International Cannabinoid Research Society (ICRS) Symposiums in 2014. I hoped that the greatest minds in cannabis science could help me understand how to use cannabis more effectively. I discovered two things during my first foray into science 1) the researchers most cited in cannabis know very little about how people use the plant *and* 2) animal studies point to therapeutic dosages in people. The year following that first conference, I began asking (hundreds of)patients how they use cannabis and how much they use. I came to find that people very clearly and naturally titrate their cannabis use to the animal study guidelines (especially when they are empowered to do so and are having success)—or they won't, but those that don't have much less success treating debilitating conditions.

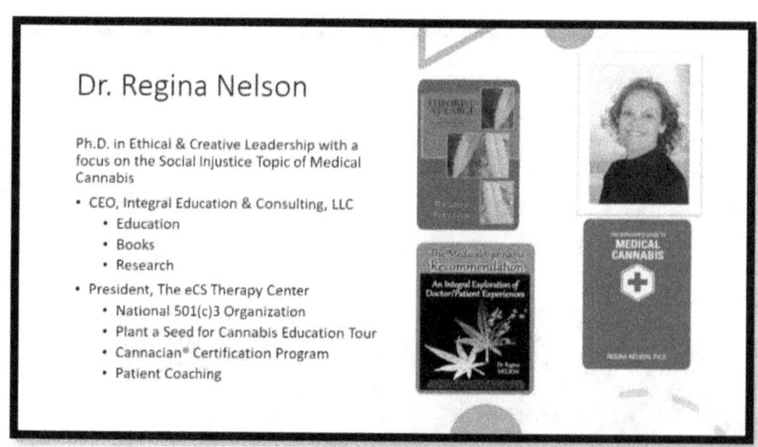

I began sharing this information widely when *The eCS Therapy Companion Guide* was published in 2015. As cannabis and the industry surrounding it continue to come out of the darkness and more people report using it medicinally we continuously learn more. I republished this title in 2018, as *The Survivor's Guide to Medical Cannabis* to include updated information, as we had learned much in just three years. Now, it is 2022, and I am about to release a second edition of *The Survivor's Guide to Medical Cannabis*. The progress in knowledge really is amazing.

The Cannacian® Level One certification covers a number of subjects that *The Survivor's Guide to Medical Cannabis* covers more thoroughly and some topics it doesn't touch on. During this session, we start by exploring "The Talk"—the talk between a doctor or a patient about medical cannabis *and* the desire for a medical cannabis recommendation. We will also discuss the endocannabinoid system (eCS) and the importance of this system to health. Next we will investigate the differences (and similarities) of hemp in contrast to cannabis. Finally, Targeted Dosing Strategies will help you put the pieces together and develop a cannabis therapy plan.

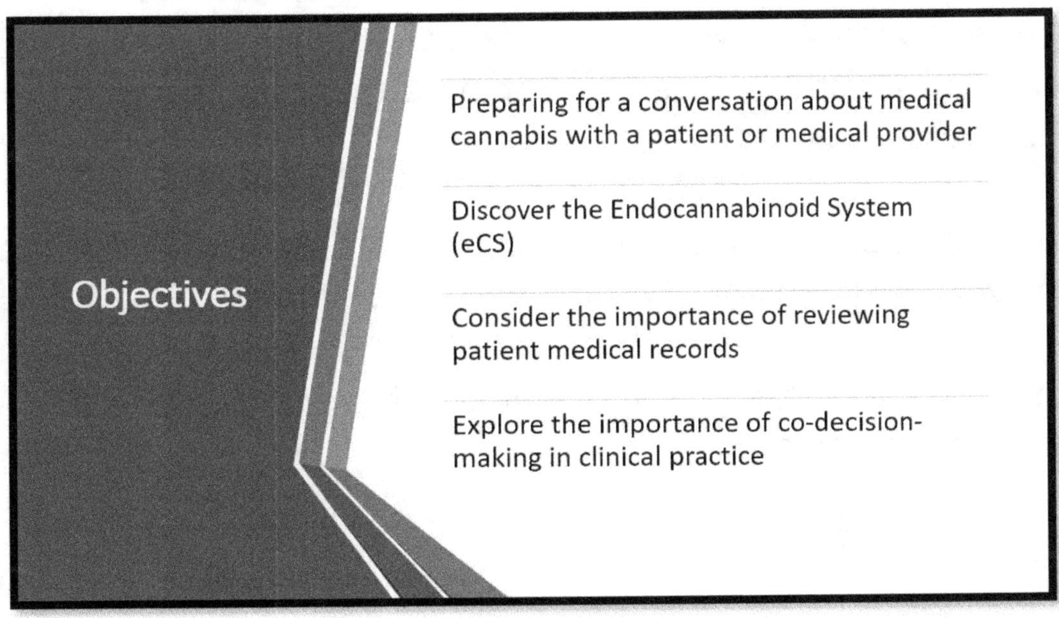

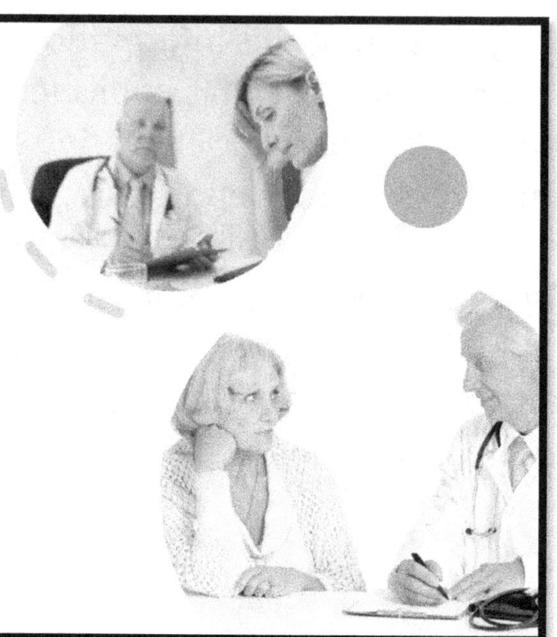

Communicating for Co-Decision Making

It's typical for the doctor to take the lead and the patient to follow. But in good patient-doctor relationships, communication is valued and a partnership in health is sought.

Patients want to be heard and the key to hearing someone is listening. Even if a doctor cannot or will not write a medical cannabis recommendation for the patient, they can listen to why the patient thinks cannabis might be a solution. Plus, the doctor should follow and track the patient's progress. Is the patient responding as well as s/he claims? Is cannabis use affecting prescription usage? (I guarantee that cannabis will impact prescription usage).

Patients must be reminded that you <u>and</u> your physician work as a team to solve *your* medical problems.

Since every human being has an *endocannabinoid system*, this conversation is important!

Why this conversation?

Endocannabinoids and their receptors are found throughout the body: in the brain, organs, connective tissues, glands, and immune cells.

The eCS is responsible for multifaceted actions in our immune system, nervous system, and all of the body's organs; *it is literally a bridge between our body and mind*.

The eCS (endocannabinoid system) has a primary purpose of keeping the body in **homeostasis**.

All of our body's natural signaling systems fluctuate, sometimes our hormones run high and sometimes low; the same with many types of brain to body and body to brain messaging. Illness or injury causes imbalance or a break in homeostasis. Suddenly your body has needs it didn't have before—long term illness may be caused by or can cause messaging errors within various bodily systems. In healing it is the job of the eCS to bring the body back to homeostasis and into balance.

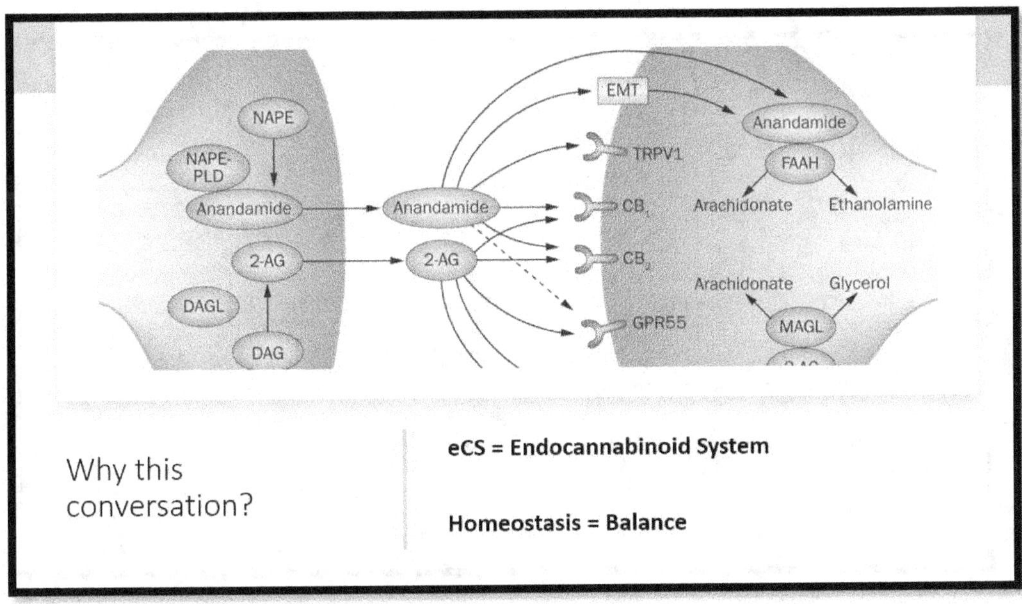

Why this
conversation?

eCS = Endocannabinoid System

Homeostasis = Balance

Preparing for "The Talk"

Patients need to prepare for the Talk (cannabis conversation) with their doctor. Doctors need to be prepared to have these talks (often).

Good preparation helps the patient assure they are speaking not from an emotional point-of-view, but from a factual one. Doctors are not prone to changing their minds about a topic as controversial as cannabis because of patient emotions. But they will listen and learn from a patient that can describe their symptoms and how cannabis can or may help alleviate them.

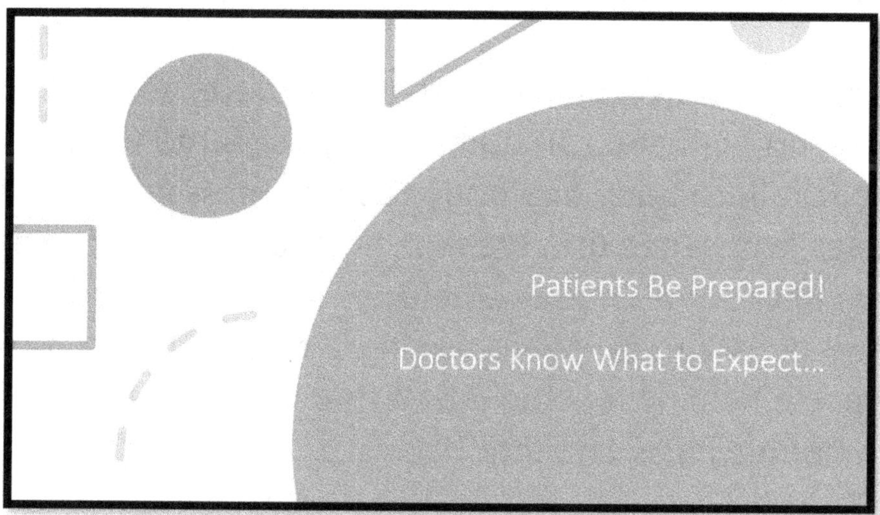

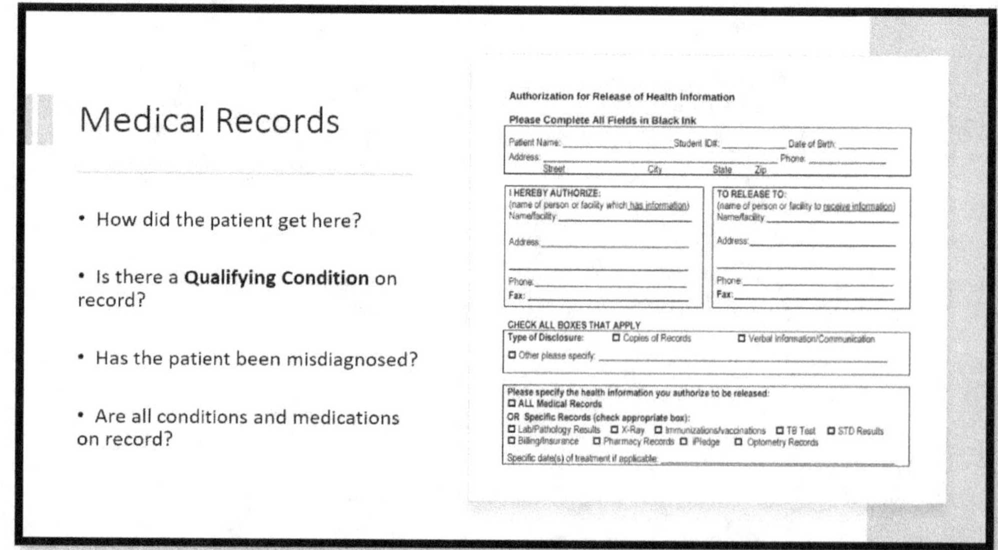

Authorization for Release of Health Information

Please Complete All Fields in Black Ink

Patient Name: _______________ Student ID#: _________ Date of Birth: _________
Address: _______________ Phone: _________
Street   City   State   Zip

I HEREBY AUTHORIZE: (name of person or facility which has information) Name/facility _______________	TO RELEASE TO: (name of person or facility to receive information) Name/facility _______________
Address: _______________	Address: _______________
Phone: _______________ Fax: _______________	Phone: _______________ Fax: _______________

CHECK ALL BOXES THAT APPLY

Type of Disclosure: ☐ Copies of Records   ☐ Verbal Information/Communication
☐ Other please specify _______________

Please specify the health information you authorize to be released:
☐ ALL Medical Records
OR Specific Records (check appropriate box):
☐ Lab/Pathology Results ☐ X-Ray ☐ Immunizations/vaccinations ☐ TB Test ☐ STD Results
☐ Billing/Insurance ☐ Pharmacy Records ☐ iPledge ☐ Optometry Records

Specific date(s) of treatment if applicable: _______________

Patients are strongly encouraged to order and review their personal medical records. You have a right to copies of any and all medical records.

Frequently patients identify incorrect or slandering information in their medical records (i.e., incorrect diagnosis(es), comments they are addicted to marijuana by personal physicians, etc.).

However, if the patient's personal doctor refuses to recommend medical cannabis and it's still an option the patient would like to pursue; having a full copy of one's medical records will help in obtaining a recommendation from a cannabis evaluation center or an Integrative Cannabis Physician.

Notes

____

____

____

____

____

____

____

____

____

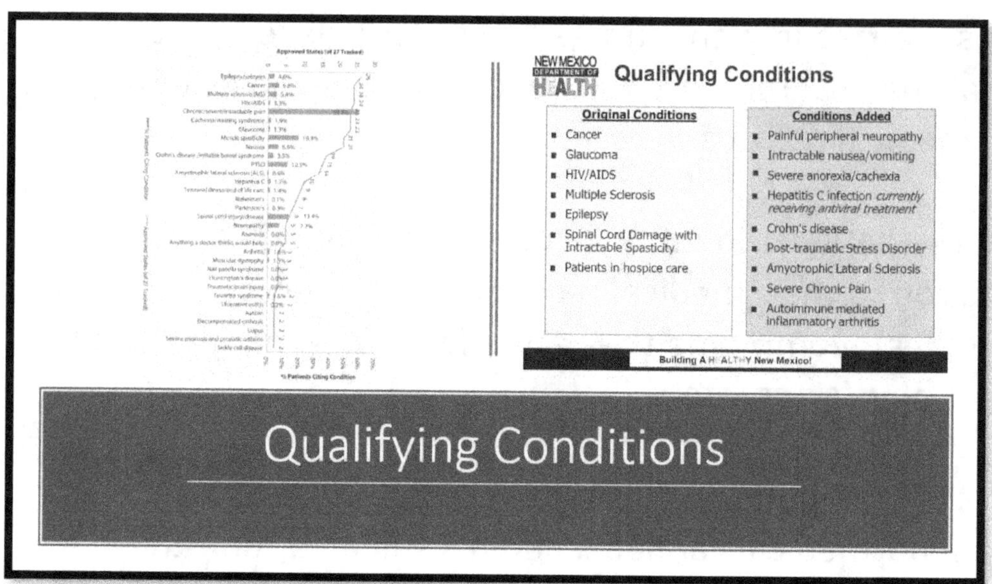

Qualifying Conditions

Medical cannabis regulations differ in every state that has an approved program (currently 37 U.S. States have some sort of medical marijuana program).

Until recently, California was the ONLY state with the 'qualifying condition' that allows "any condition that a physician believes cannabis may provide benefit" to be used. In 2018,Oklahoma implemented SQ788, which also allows a physician to recommend for any condition -- and the law does not specify *any* specific qualifying conditions. While this was a bold move, it does much to acknowledge that all humans have an eCS. Cannabis may be helpful to many, if not nearly all, conditions from which we humans suffer.

Remember we all have an eCS!

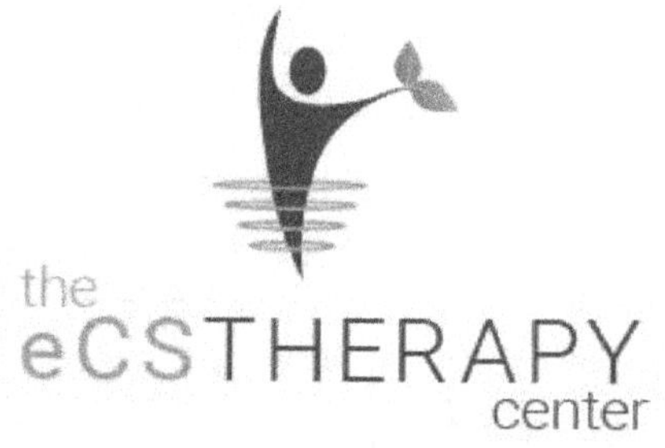

Qualifying Medical Conditions

Before engaging in a conversation about cannabis with a doctor, a patient should make a list of their qualifying condition(s) and symptoms, include a description of symptoms on their *worst* day, *and* all treatments that have been attempted.

It is also important to list the side-effects the patient experienced from conventional medical treatment. By reviewing the patient's records one can assure they meet the guidelines set by the state before approaching a primary or specialty physicians for a recommendation.

A medical cannabis recommendation is a verification, signed by a physician, that you have a 'qualifying diagnosis' and meet the requirements of the state's medical marijuana program.

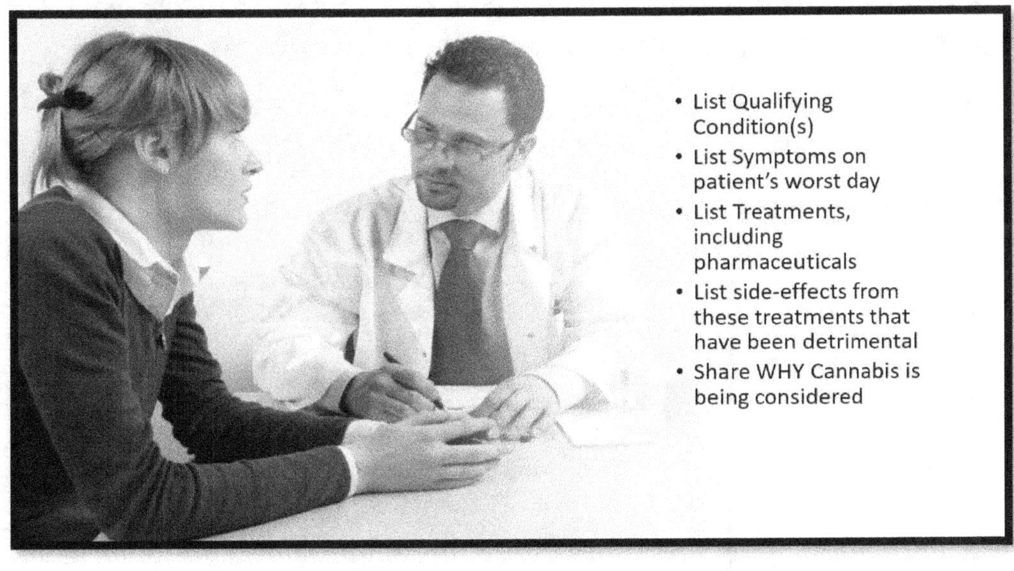

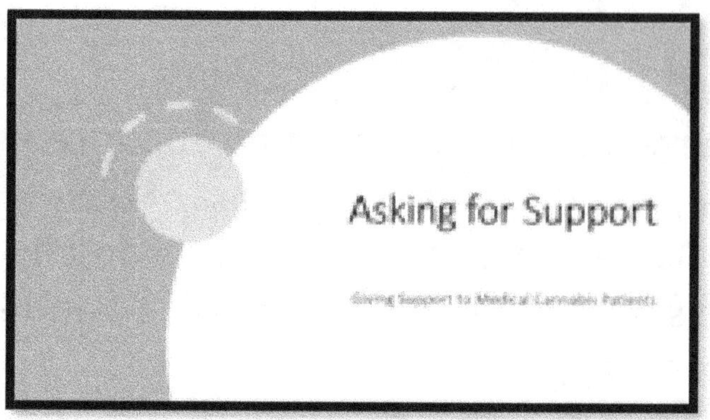

Honest Communication

A patient meeting with a doctor for a medical cannabis recommendation should be honest about their health by sharing their medical experience (and records) with the physician.

The patient should be prepared to explain to the doctor how you've responded to prescribed medications and the side-effects you've endured. The physician should also be informed about what's worked for the patient and why specifically medical cannabis might be a good solution.

If the patient is currently using cannabis or has tried cannabis to see if it might work for them, they should honestly describe when they began treating with cannabis, the amount of cannabis they use, how often and by what delivery methods. Patients can also the importance of accessing a safe, standardized, legal supply of medical cannabis.

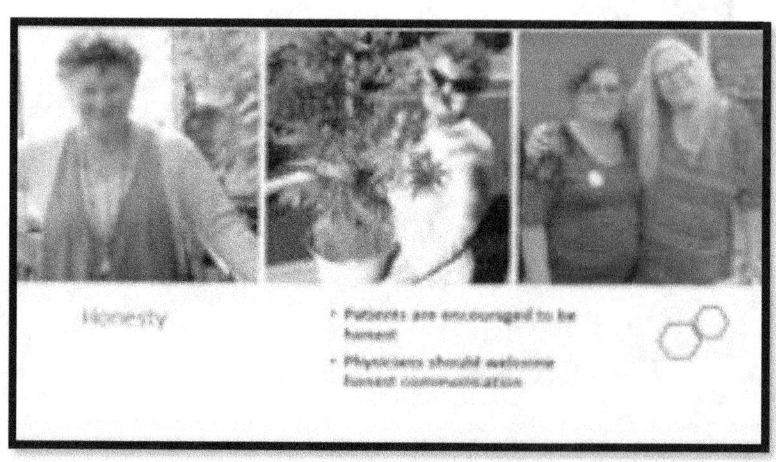

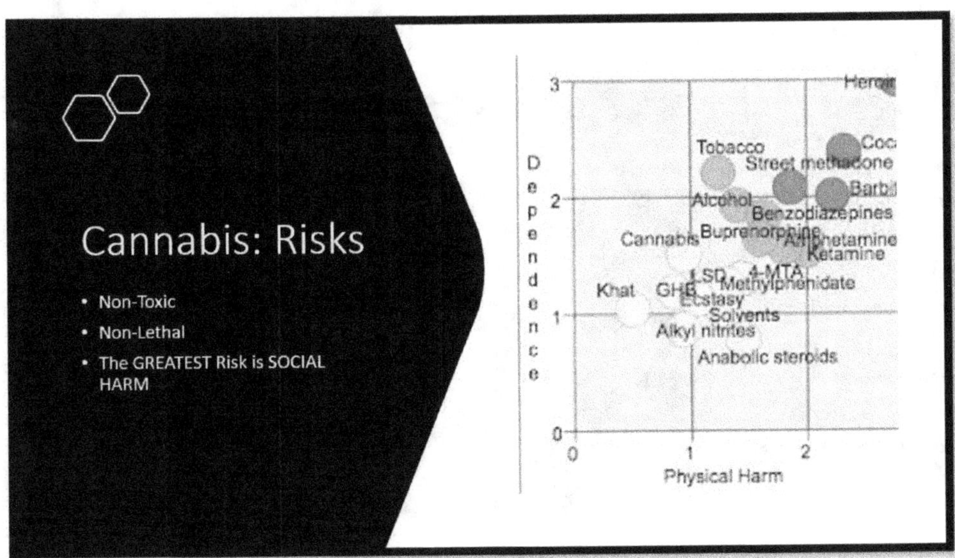

Cannabis and Safety in Humans

Despite the fact that significant scientific evidence shows that cannabis is non-toxic, free of harmful side-effects, is neurogenerative, neuroprotective, and every human being has an endocannabinoid system -- we cannot lose sight of the fact that *cannabis sativa* remains a Schedule One drug -- which means it is classified as being highly dangerous, highly addictive and non-medicinal.

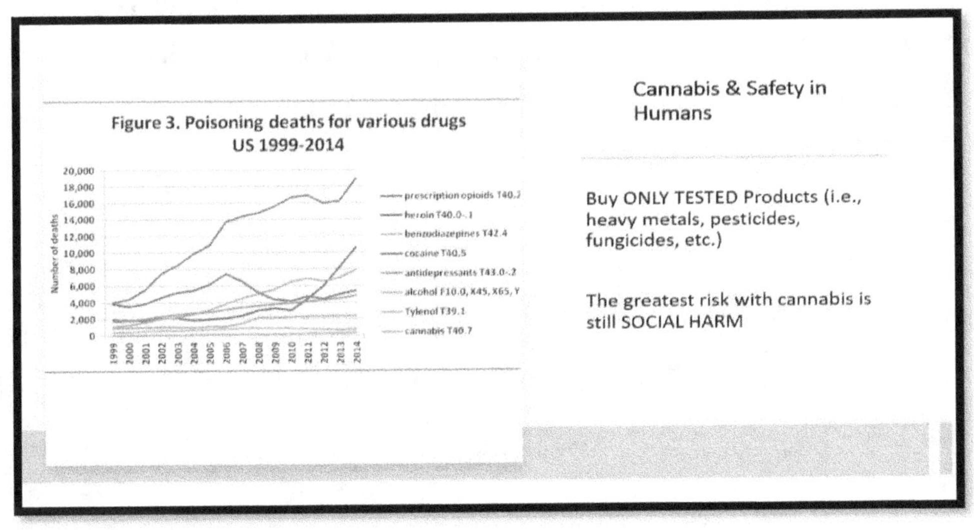

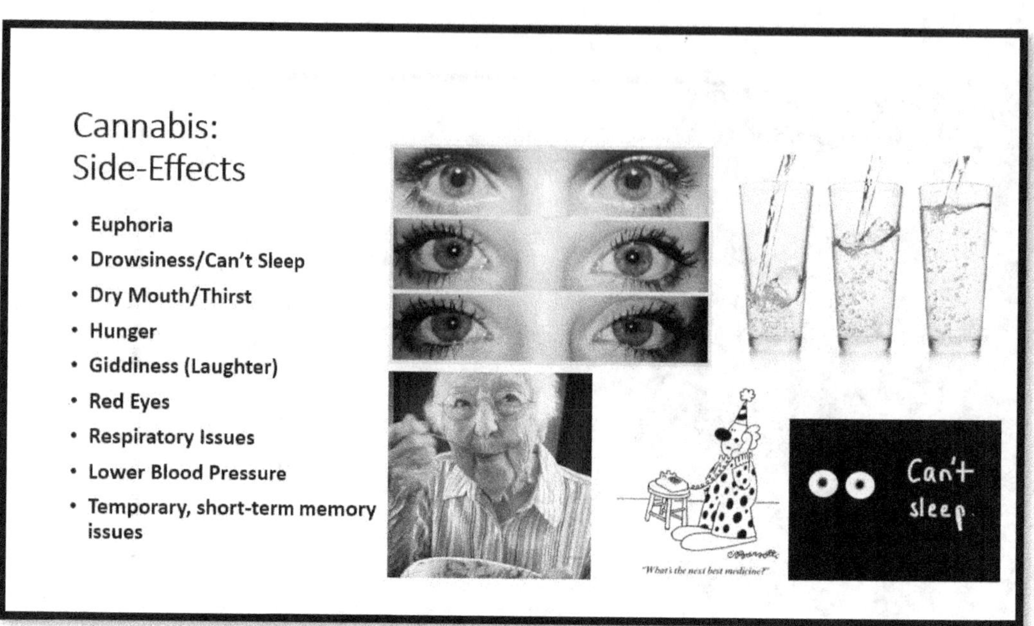

Cannabis: Side-Effects

Euphoria

The euphoric experience associated with cannabis, and specifically the cannabinoid THC, is at the center of social stigma surrounding cannabis use. Yet, for the chronic and terminally ill the euphoric side effect can be hugely beneficial.

Medical cannabis patients are not 'high-seekers' in the sense that they're addicted and only want more euphoria. Instead, the immediate release of stress and relaxation of tension that accompany THC's euphoric effects may often be greatly welcomed by the chronically and terminally ill.

A Question to Ponder
Why is the euphoric effect of cannabis socially stigmatized?

Drowsiness – Insomnia

Primarily strain specific (I.e., terpene specific). but it can also be dose related.

Dry Mouth or Thirst

A well-known side-effect that can be combated with water.

Giddiness

Laughter that becomes uncontrollable, or nearly so, can be good for those who've been ill for quite some time. Plus, even studies show that fake laughter has positive health effects.

Hunger

Studies show, and users know cannabis impacts appetite (the 'munchies' have the added effected of making food taste and smell better too). However, studies also shown that cannabis users have leaner frames than non-cannabis users. In fact, many patients report weight loss after engaging in a cannabis regime—feeling better, getting more active, and eating more consciously are also widely reported side-effects of cannabis use.

Red Eyes

This effect is due to vascular dilation—the blood vessels in the eyes enlarge and the eyes get red and dilate. This side-effect is temporary.

Respiratory Issues

Respiratory issues are most frequently caused by patients smoking moldy or mildew-ridden cannabis products, not from the cannabis itself. Studies show the most prominent effect from smoking cannabis is an enlarged lung capacity, as cannabis is a bronchial dilator.

Temporary, Short-Term Memory Loss

A side-effect of euphoria is short-term, temporary memory loss. Like, 'where did I put my phone?' But over an extended period of time cannabis use actually improves memory.

Uneasiness or Anxiety

Often caused by 'sativa' strains (I.e., terpenes) but may also be due to THC-sensitivity or from ingesting too much cannabis.

You can have a very unpleasant or even distressing experience caused by over consuming cannabis.

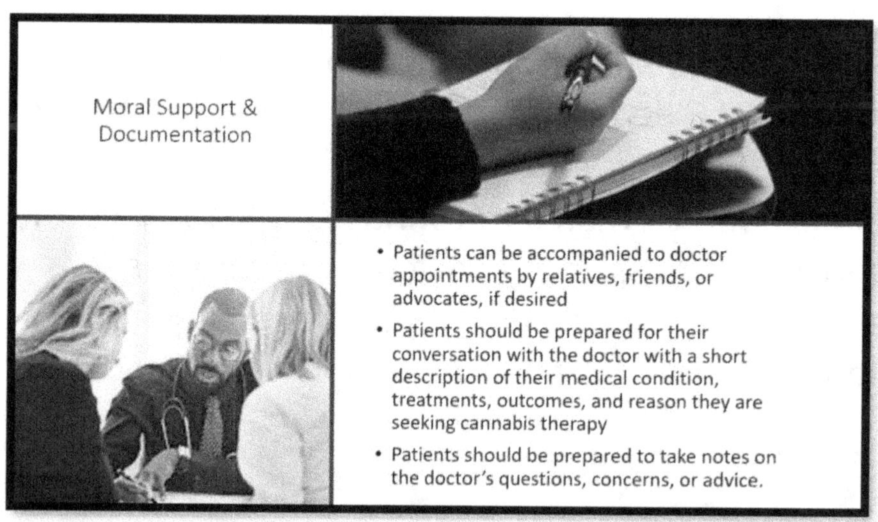

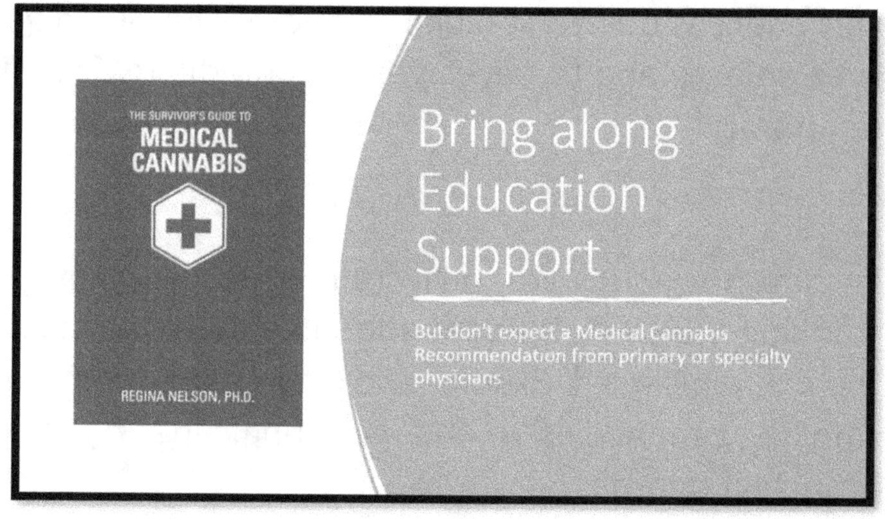

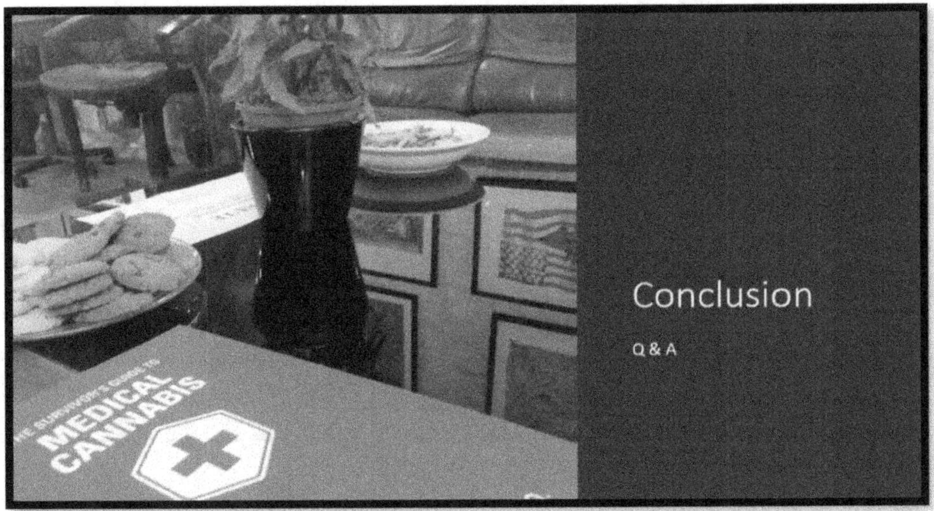

Notes

____

____

____

____

____

____

____

____

____

Notes

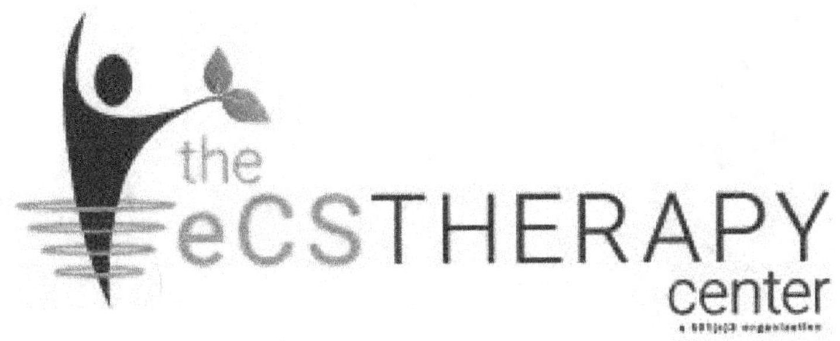

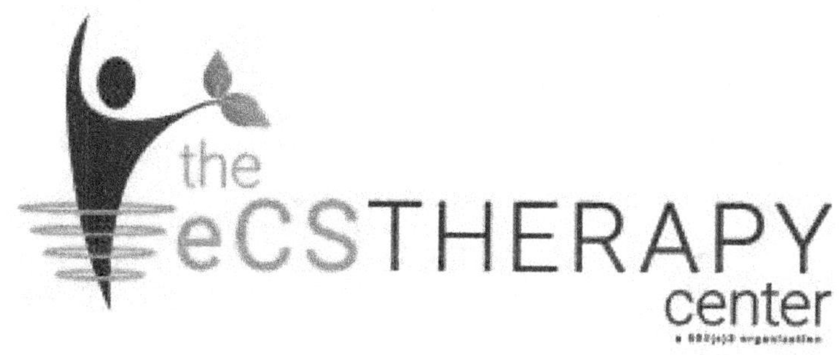

Welcome to
An Introduction to the Endocannabinoid System (eCS)

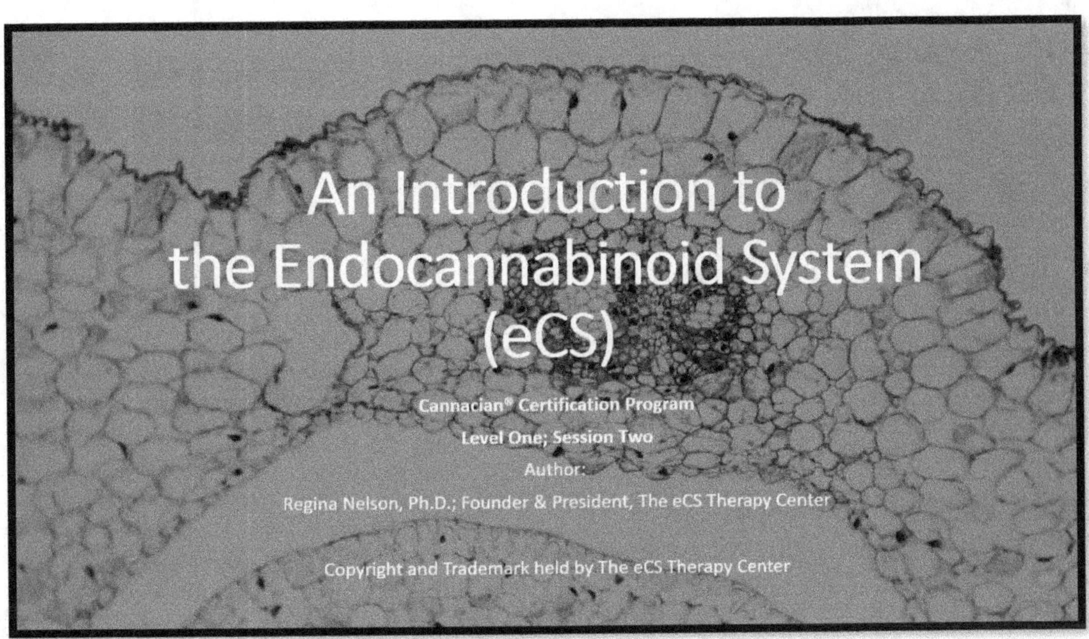

Objectives

- Assist participants in developing a basic understanding of the endocannabinoid system (eCS);
- Learn the active definitions of *cannabis sativa, cannabis indica,* and *cannabis ruderalis*
- Explore the ways phytocannabinoids interact with the eCS;
- Learn the various ways cannabis can be delivered;
- Briefly examine target dosing guidelines.

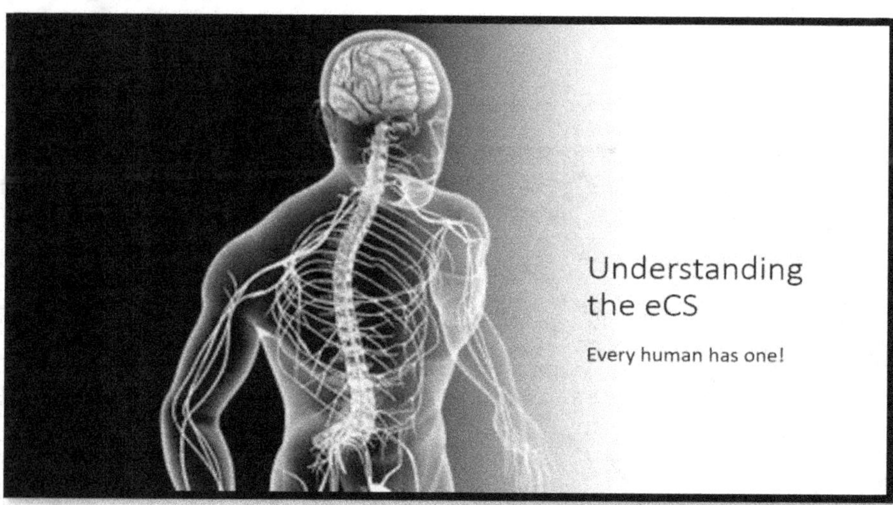

What is the eCS?

The **endocannabinoid system** (eCS) is named after the *cannabis sativa* plant that led to its discovery.

The eCS is perhaps the most important physiologic (bodily) system involved in establishing and maintaining human health.

The goal of the eCS is to bring *homeostasis*, or balance, to the human body. Throughout the human body, the endocannabinoid system performs different tasks at a cellular level.

Endogenous Cannabinoids

Endo means *within*—so endogenous cannabinoids are natural *within* our own bodies.

The eCS is an essential part of life as it allows us to adapt to environmental changes, both internal and external fluctuations in our bodily environment.

Sufficient research indicates that a properly functioning eCS is necessary for good health and that certain medical conditions may be the result of deficiencies within this system.

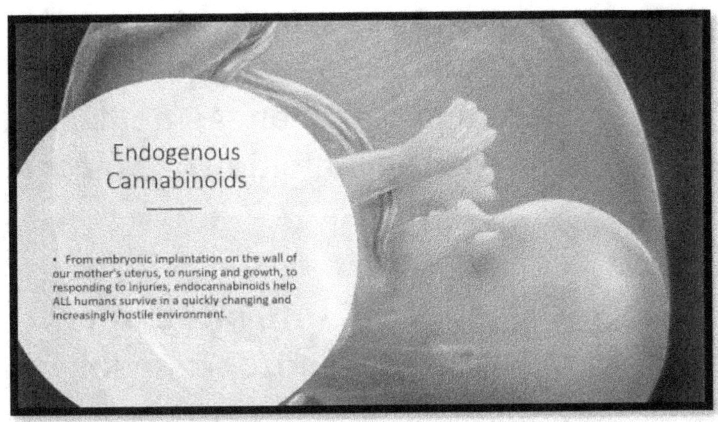

Endocannabinoids

Endocannabinoids are found at the intersection of the body's various systems. They are responsible for communication and coordination between different cell types. To date, we know the most about two types of endogenous cannabinoids: Anandamide and 2-arachidonylglycerol (2-AG).

Both are ligands or fat molecules—in that they are molecules that are produced as needed to stimulate endocannabinoid and other receptors in order to bring homeostasis to the body.

Anandamide is a neuro-transmitting lipid (fat) compound made by all mammals. It might be described as a self-manufactured or "natural THC" circulating within the body.

Both anandamide and THC act through the cannabinoid receptors and have similar effects on appetite, memory, and pau=in reception. Anandamide also has a poorly understood but important role in hormonal balance and the reproductive system. Anandamide may be is also responsible for helping us maintain good sleep patterns.

2-arachidonylglycerol or 2-AG is the most abundant endocannabinoid found in the body, and like anandamide, it is thought to play an important role in the regulation of appetite, immune system functions and pain management. Studies find that 2-AG also plays a role in the inhibition of cancer cell production.

Other recent studies suggest that 2-AG, rather than anandamide, is the true natural ligand for cannabinoid receptors and the key endocannabinoid involved in retrograde signaling in the brain (meaning it can help send and receive signals/messages throughout the body).

Endocannabinoids

Anandamide

2-Arachidonyl-glycerol (2-AG)

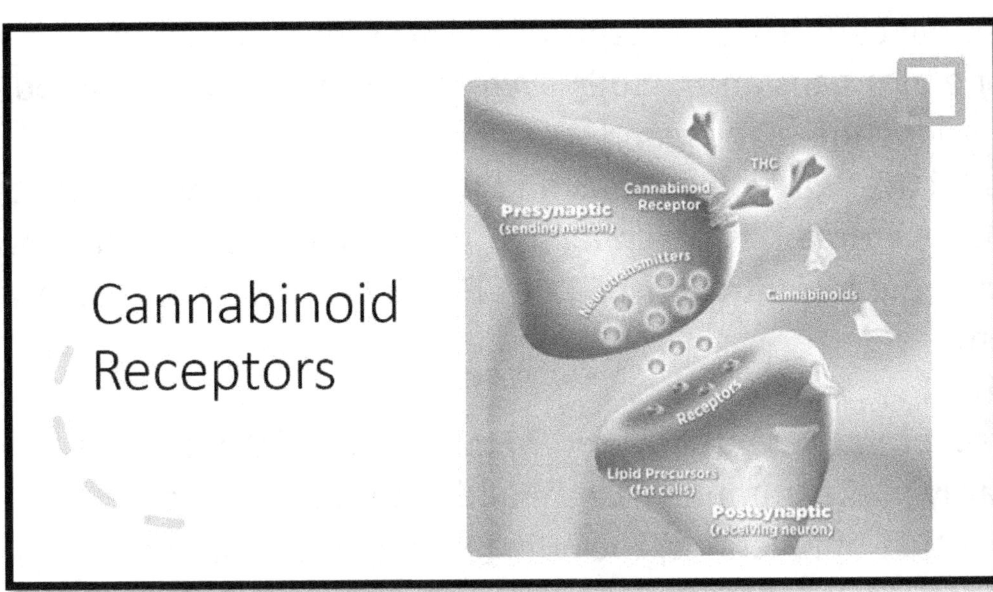

Cannabinoid Receptors

Cannabinoid receptors occur naturally – not only in humans – but in all mammals.

Cannabinoid receptor* molecules give chemical substances that transmit messages a place to act. These receptors are located primarily in the nervous system and immune system. *These receptors are important to the communication that bridge mind and body.

Endocannabinoids, anandamide and 2-AG occur naturally in the body and have effect on cannabinoid receptors, as ligands or fat messengers. *Phytocannabinoids* occur naturally within the *cannabis sativa* plant and activate or stimulate the same receptor system. In the pharmaceutical market we're also potentially exposed to *Synthetic Cannabinoids*, manmade cannabinoid doppelgangers. Synthetic cannabinoids don't have the same effect or safety profile of cannabis. Spice, K-2, and some other synthetic cannabinoids have been rightfully criminalized due to their toxic side-effects.

CB₁ receptors reside predominantly on nerve cells in the brain and spinal cord. These receptors are also found in some peripheral organs and tissues such as the spleen, white blood cells, endocrine glands, and parts of the reproductive, gastrointestinal and urinary tracts. **The stimulation of CB$_1$ receptors has psychoactive and behavioral effects even without the introduction of THC**. This is the feel-good receptor system!

CB₂ receptors were discovered in the early 1990s; these reside primarily in the immune system and are involved in the modulation of functions, including inflammation and pain response. CB$_2$ receptors are mainly found on white blood cells, in the tonsils, and in the spleen. Immune cells express far more CB$_2$ receptors than CB$_1$ receptors though both are present.

Notes

____

____

____

____

____

____

____

____

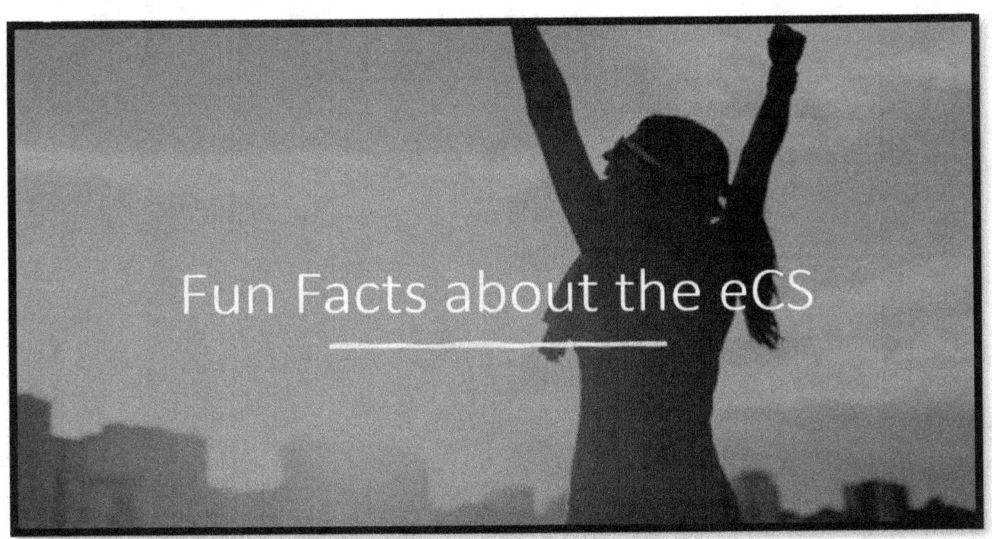

Fun Facts about the eCS and Cannabinoids

Anandamide is a self-manufactured "natural THC" circulating within the body. It increases in a woman upon the birth of a child and as she begins expressing it into her breast milk. The same chemical that causes the munchies in adults, helps a newborn baby seek to suckle and nourish itself.

Anandamide was named by the discovering team of scientists led by Dr. Raphael Mechoulam in 1992. The word combines the Sanskrit word, 'ananda' meaning "bliss" and 'amide' meaning 'chemical type' —a solid description given how similarly it works to cannabinoid THC within the body.

Anandamide is now understood as the source of the runner's high. Anandamide has also been found in chocolate - its presence may be partly responsible for the enjoyment many of us experience while eating it. This is the reason some people feel 'euphoric' when eating chocolate (i.e., spicy food rich in capsaicin may also be responsible for this type of reaction).

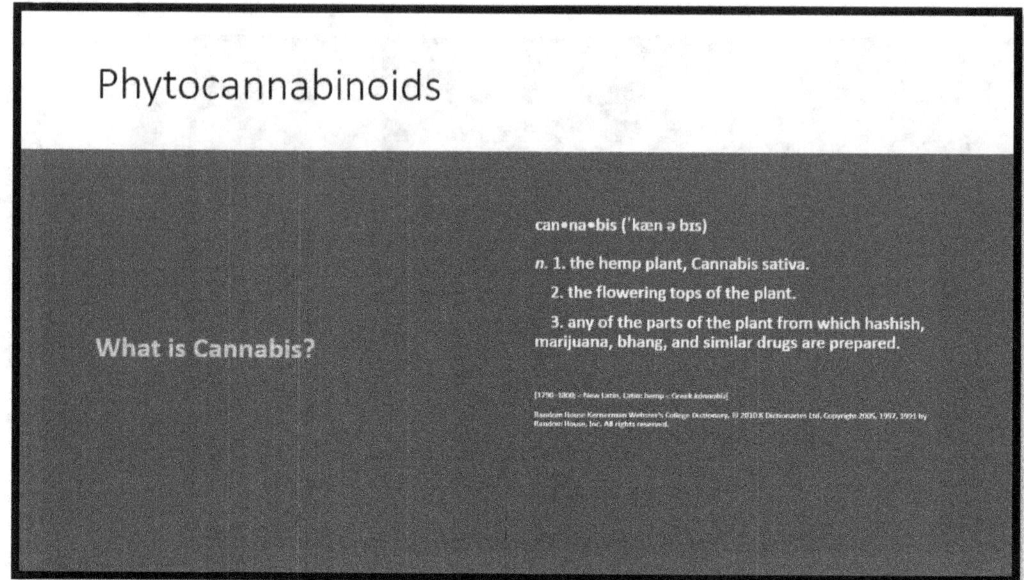

Phytocannabinoids

Phytocannabinoids are simply the cannabinoids that are endogenous (within) to the *cannabis sativa* plant.

As we think about the plant now in the cannabis industry, we define the *cannabis sativa* plant in these three (3) categories, as we will discuss in Hemp v Cannabis, these definitions aren't correct, but they are common, so patients should understand theterms.

cannabis sativa (which tends to provide terpenes that give alertness or energy to the patient)

cannabis indica (which tends to provide terpenes that allow the patient to relax and rest)

cannabis ruderalis (is more commonly known as hemp—and hemp can have a significant amount of cannabinoids or it can have hardly any, depending on the strain. Though many hemp strains have few cannabinoids, they do have other industrial uses besides medicine.

As we discussed in the "Time for the Talk" Module—Cannabis is non-toxic. I like to think of it along the lines of crayons— Crayons are non-toxic, but if your child eats a whole box of crayons, she very well may get sick, BUT she won't die (and remember, crayons had to be regulated to become non-toxic after children died from eating them).

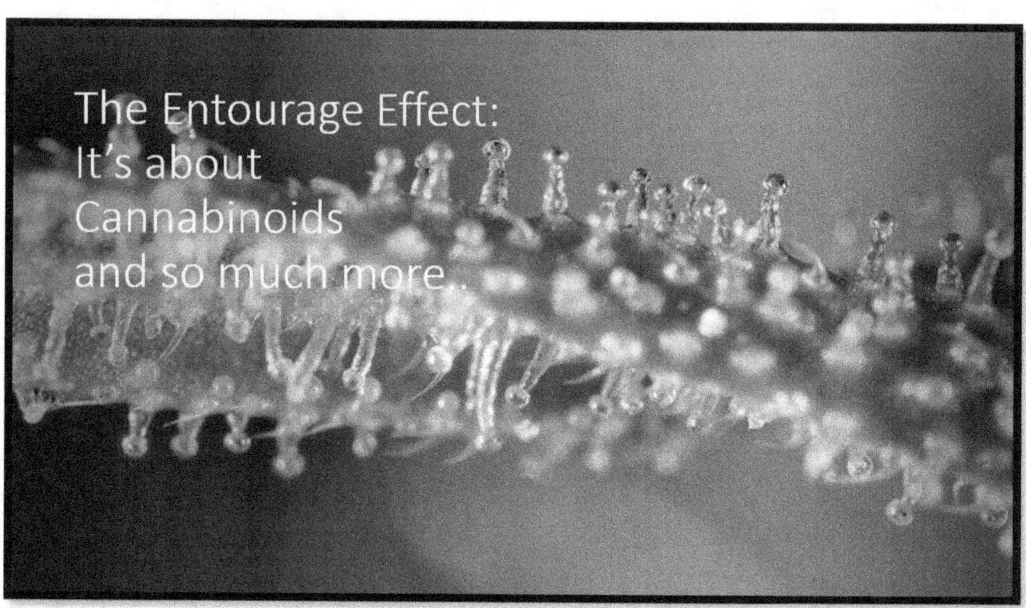

The Entourage Effect

Cannabis sativa contains over 420 different chemical compounds, including over 60 cannabinoids. Cannabinoid plant chemistry is far more complex than that of THC, as a singular cannabinoid of interest. Different effects may be experienced due to the presence of additional cannabinoids and other compounds. Eighteen different classes of chemicals including nitrogenous compounds, amino acids, hydrocarbons, carbohydrates, terpenes, and simple and fatty acids, contribute to the known pharmacological and toxicological properties of cannabis. We won't be discussing them all in this program, but it is important to recognize cannabis is a complex plant.

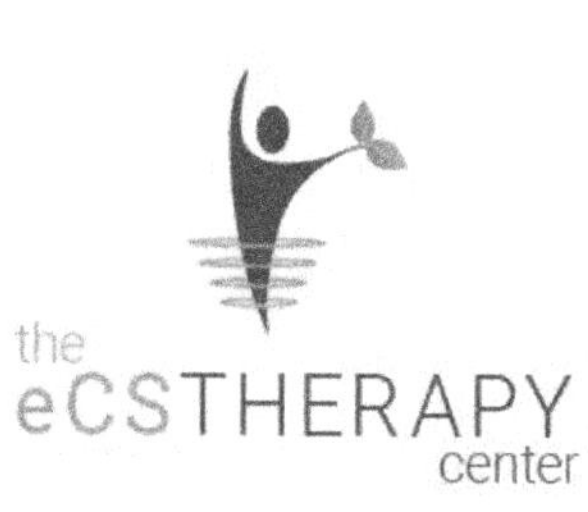

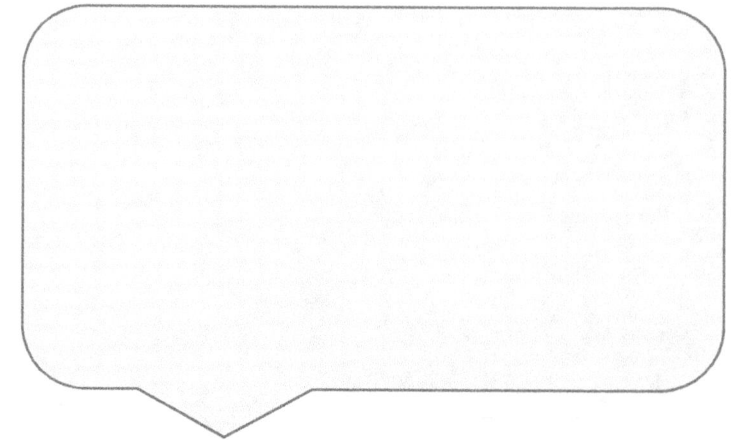

T.H.C. or delta-9-tetrahydrocannabinol

The most recognized and notorious cannabinoid is *delta-9-tetrahydrocannabinol*. THC has the most significant psychoactive effect of the cannabinoids; thus, it has mostly been studied as a drug of abuse.

The ratio of THC to other cannabinoids varies from strain-to-strain as does the experienced psychoactive experience, since some cannabinoids like CBD appear to mitigate THC's euphoric effects.

For example, at an 8:1 ratio of CBD:THC people rarely report 'feeling' any euphoric side-effects (though they may report relaxation, stress-relief, sleep, etc., which technically are psychoactive effects).

THC is known to provide some of the following therapeutic effects: muscle relaxant, anti-cancer, anti-epileptic, anti-emetic, anti-inflammatory, appetite stimulating, bronchodilation, hypotension, anti-depressant and analgesic (pain relief) effects.

Δ9-Tetrahydrocannabinol (T.H.C.)

CO_2

Decarboxylation (Loss of CO_2)

CO_2

THCA

THC

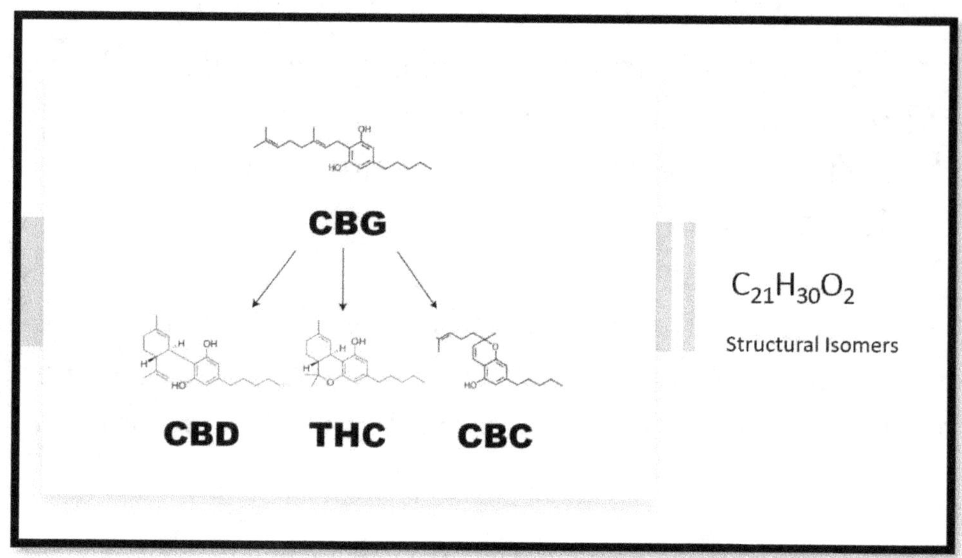

As we move forward to discuss the second most talked about cannabinoid, CBD, it's important to note that in chemistry terms THC, CBD, and CBC are known as *structural isomers*: they are each 21-carbon containing phytocannabinoids, which share an identical chemical formula, $C_{21}H_{30}O_2$. However, the atoms are arranged slightly different in the molecules. For example, the key structural difference between THC and CBD is an oxygen-containing closed ring in THC molecules, which is open in CBD molecules.

Notes

____

____

____

____

____

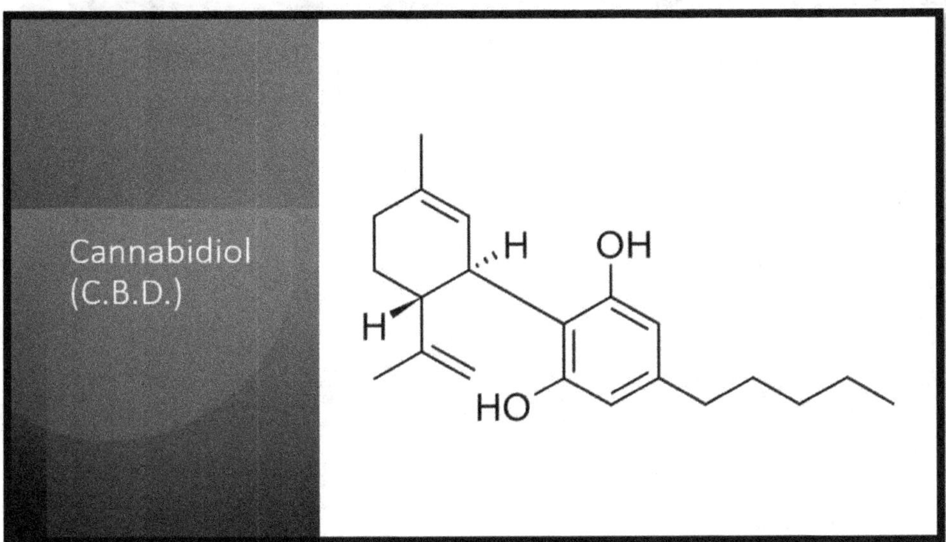

Cannabidiol or C.B.D.

Generally, cannabidiol or C.B.D. appears to be neuroprotective; which means that it may prevent as well as keep neurological disease (or injury) from progressing. In addition, it also positively effects inflammation, anxiety, and nausea. CND has many of the same therapeutic qualities as THC, but with significantly less euphoric power of its own.

There is no doubt that CBD is an extremely important cannabinoid and its therapeutic potential is enormous. CBD holds the potential to treat dozens of serious and life-threatening conditions, including Parkinson's disease, Alzheimer's disease, cerebral ischemia, diabetes, rheumatoid arthritis, other inflammatory diseases, nausea, and cancer, and as the media in America is following it often works miracles in epileptic seizures, again particularly those with Dravet's Syndrome.

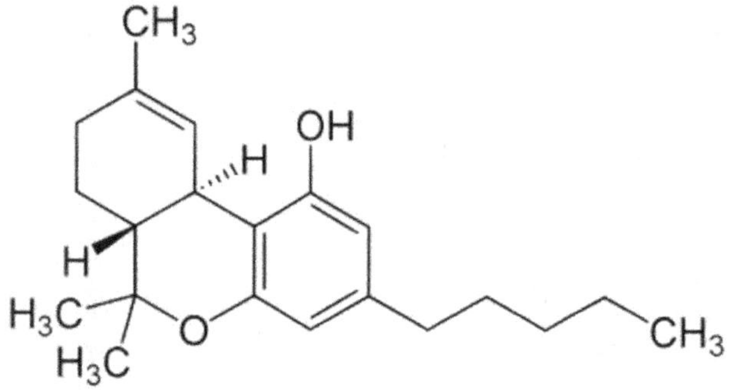

Cannabinol or C.B.N.

Cannabinol is largely a product of THC deterioration because it is a derivative of THC. CBN is found in large concentrations of cannabis oil that's been scorched or heated to the point the THC has degraded into CBN, and cannabis that has been improperly stored for long periods of time (think, Mexican Cartel 'brick weed').

CBD tinctures (particularly those on the medical cannabis market) often have a significant content of CBN, meaning the THC has been scorched and turned to CBN.

Compared with THC, CBN binds relatively weakly with the body's endogenous cannabinoid receptors. But CBN is rightfully blamed for the 'couch-lock' side-effect often associated with cannabis use, as CBN has a sedative effect.

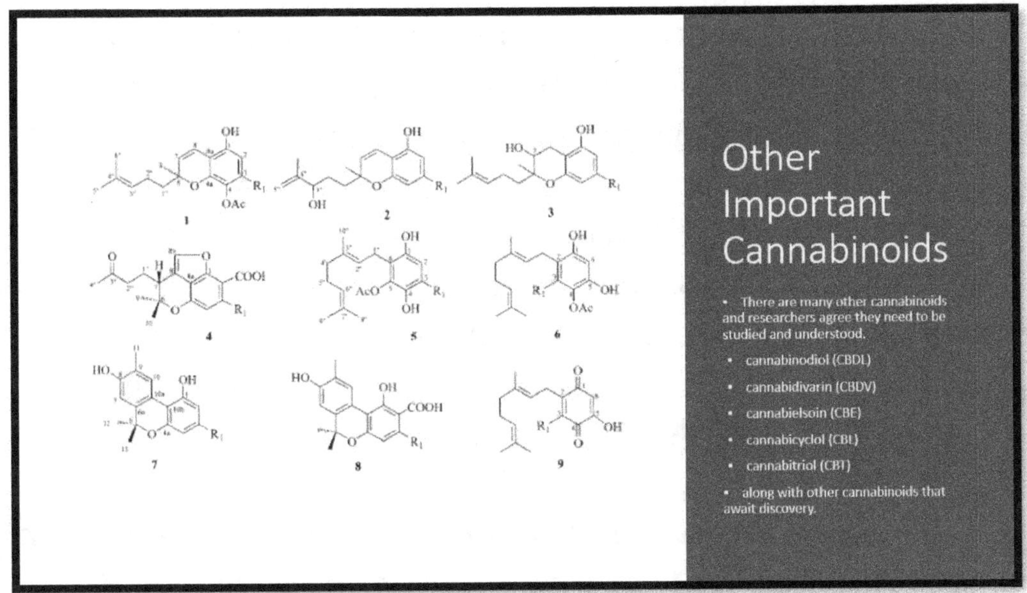

Other Important Cannabinoids

- There are many other cannabinoids and researchers agree they need to be studied and understood.
- cannabinodiol (CBDL)
- cannabidivarin (CBDV)
- cannabielsoin (CBE)
- cannabicyclol (CBL)
- cannabitriol (CBT)
- along with other cannabinoids that await discovery.

Beyond the Smoke: Delivery Methods

Smoking Cannabis

Smoking cannabis is very much considered *recreational* use by medical professionals and the public in general. As you may have noticed I have avoided the term 'recreational'. Dr. Allen Frankel and I were chatting about the importance of language when he mentioned he's switched his vernacular to "casual vs. recreational" and "focused vs. medical" uses of cannabis. This terminology has resonated well with me and I hope it does with you as well, because 'recreational' use is stigmatized and considered 'bad' because of prohibition.

Might it be possible that many people have been searching to fill a void or deficiency that they could not quite explain? Perhaps, an endocannabinoid deficiency?

Smoking cannabis delivers active cannabinoids within seconds. Medicine is absorbed in the lungs and begins circulating in the blood stream immediately, breaking the blood/brain barrier within seconds (fat ligands have no trouble breaking this barrier, signaling, and/or developing receptors in the brain).

Since the effects of inhaled cannabis are rapid, it is easy for patients to titrate their dose by simply waiting a few minutes in between inhalations. For pain issues, muscle spasm or stiffness, or nausea, for example, instead of reaching for an over-the-counter pain reliever or prescription, cannabis is often helpful as a first line of treatment.

Recent studies show no long-term damage to cannabis user's lungs even after more than 40 years of cannabis use, primarily ingested via smoking. Cannabis users show an increased lung capacity that is noteworthy (i.e., think about how holding in a bong-hit might expand the lungs), but overall the people studied had no ill effects from smoking cannabis.

Assuring one's medicine is free of mold and mildew (especially in an illegal market, and even when purchased legally in dispensaries) is vital. For those with respiratory issues—and even those without—vaporizing is recommended.

Cannabis is a natural bronchodilator and vasodilator. I've often been told by patients that vaporizing cannabis is more effective than albuterol treatments via nebulizer. Given how often I've heard this description, this is how I've begun explaining the vapor delivery process - it just makes sense given the therapeutic response.

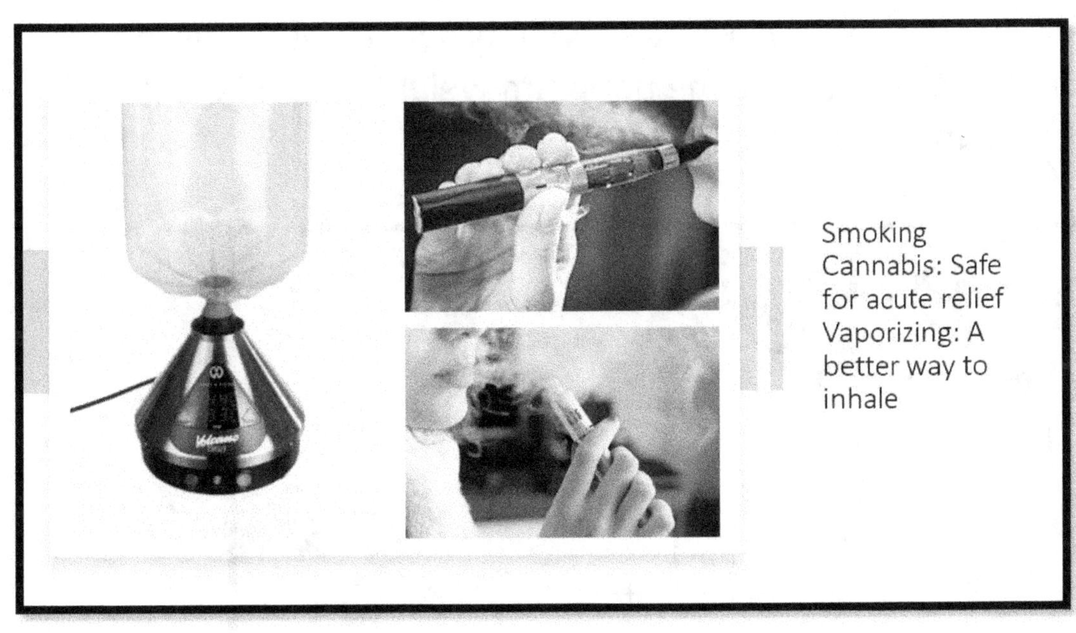

Smoking Cannabis: Safe for acute relief
Vaporizing: A better way to inhale

Cannabis Concentrates

Hash (hashish) is simply resin collected from the flowers of the cannabis plant. The primary active substance is THC, although other cannabinoids and compounds are also present. Hash is a cannabis concentrate with a long history of use because it's simple to make and it has a grand euphoric effect.--and it is great for pain control. Though hash is often smoked or vaporized it is also frequently put into capsules and used orally. This is because it's easy to dose by measured weight (1 gram of hash = approx. 700-800 mg of cannabinoids).

There is little difference between **essential oil, shatter and wax** other than the consistency, EXCEPT for in how it's made—from butane extractions, CO_2 extractions, or alcohol (grain alcohol) extractions. From a patient perspective it is vital to be assured that all solvents have been appropriately purged from the final product. There are many different processes used to make these highly potent extracts. At the end of the day it all comes down to the filtering and purging process that produces the varying products: essential oil, shatter, or wax. 1000 mg per gram weight, 600-800 mg cannabinoids by weight.

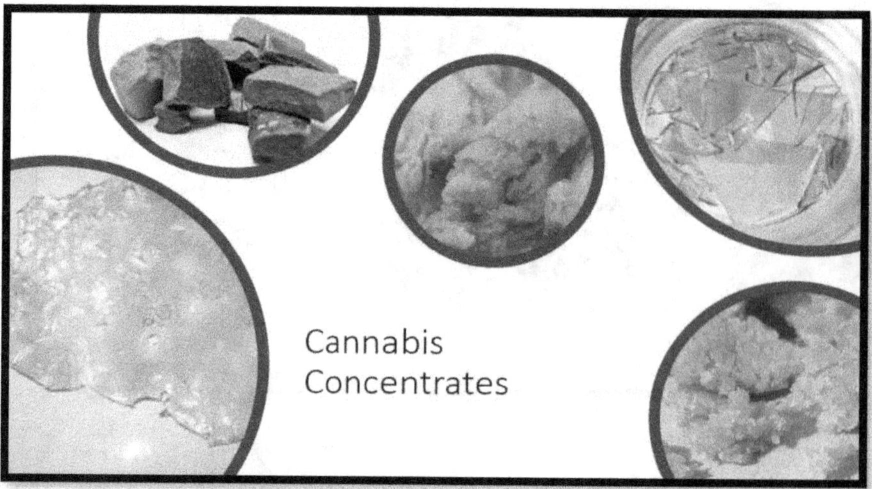

Cannabis Oil (FECO or CO)

Years of observing patients and listening to their experiences using cannabis oils has solidified my opinion that serious health issues respond more favorably with full extract cannabis oil (FECO) than with extractions that do not contain as full a cannabinoid profile.

The essential oil of the plant simply extracted with food-grade grain alcohol (like EverClear) is perhaps the best medicinal option from this miraculous plant (with juicing being a closely competing method but less available for access). The *essential oil offers the easiest dosing options because it can be the base of nearly any cannabis product (put it in capsules, include it in edibles, make suppositories, etc.).*

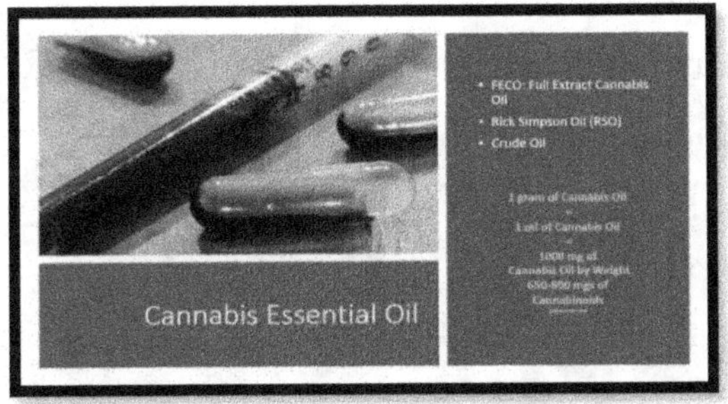

FECO is also known as cannabis oil, Rick Simpson Oil (RSO), or Phoenix Tears. It is a dark green (or amber), thick essential oil consisting of concentrated cannabinoids from the flowers and leaves of the cannabis plant. Making cannabis oil requires extraction of the cannabinoids from plant matter with a solvent, sometimes cooking to decarboxylate the cannabinoids and sometimes not (cold extraction), but solvents should be fully purged from the final product.

Over the course of time, ingesting small amounts of cannabis oil will fail to bring the same euphoric effects as those experienced as a new cannabis user. As the cannabinoids build and store within the body the body becomes less responsive to the psychoactive effects that can be unpleasant to new users. More experienced users, like myself, we miss these effects, but still receive symptom relief.

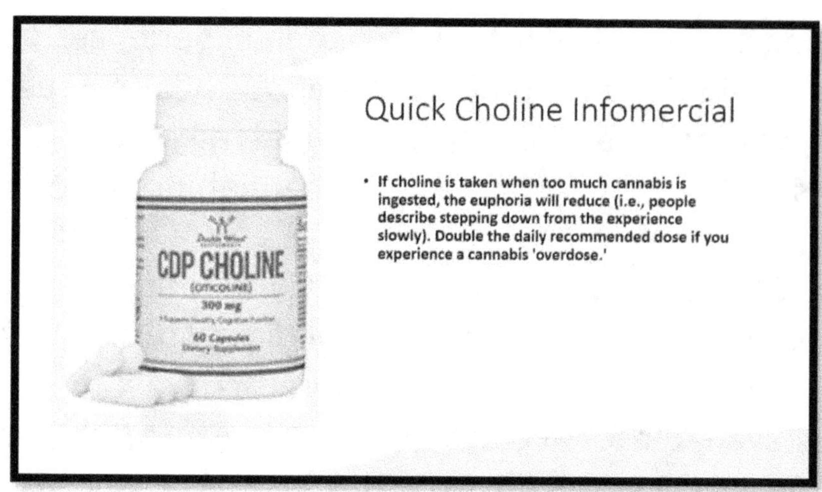

Quick Choline Infomercial

Choline supplements increase the body's natural acetylcholine. Part of what causes the 'high' sensation or euphoria is a drop-in acetylcholine levels.

By increasing the acetylcholine levels BEFORE using cannabis, less euphoria results.

Also, if taken when too much cannabis is ingested, the euphoria will reduce (i.e., people describe stepping down from the experience slowly).

That all said, people should seek a GDP Choline. Patients with brain cancer should avoid choline supplements. (The pix shown are just a visual example, they are NOT a recommendation as to brand).

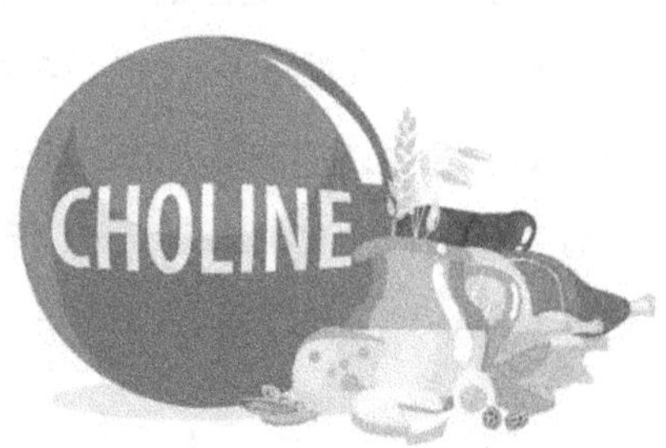

Notes

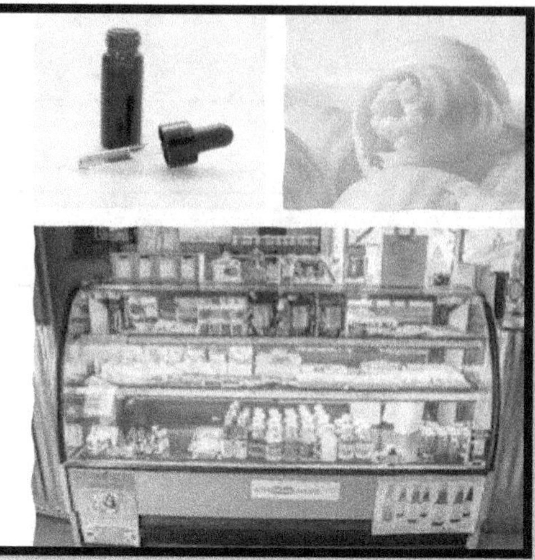

Sublingual or Edible?

Tinctures

Tinctures are great beginning treatment option for those new to cannabis or those needing to slowly increase their cannabinoid intake.

The benefit from smoking as a route of administration is rapid action and the ability of the patient to self-titrate the dose needed for relief. With tinctures patients can achieve similar rapid relief and the ability to control dose. Tinctures are not new; until cannabis was criminalized, tinctures were the primary type of cannabis medicine.

Tinctures are a rapid medicine delivery system if used sublingually and help provide consistent dosing. Titration or dose control is easily achieved by the number of drops a patient places under the tongue. Patients new to cannabis therapy can start with a small dose by using just one drop, wait for the desired medical effects (at least 15 minutes), and either increase the dose or consider the dose achieved, as the embodied experience indicates.

In addition to tinctures, suspensions are a popular product and easy to dose. For pediatric patients and adults new to cannabis therapy suspensions provide a diluted means in which cannabis oil (typically, FECO or another concentrate) can be appropriately dosed at very low levels. Some patients prefer suspensions made with coconut oil, others honey or sesame oil, but primarily when dealing with pediatric patients or those with sensitive gastric systems, olive oil is recommended.

Foods infused with cannabis are excellent for dosing throughout the day, but they're very different from smoking or tinctures in that they must pass through our digestive system. For this reason, they DO NOT provide rapid relief—instead more of a slow, extended relief.

Note: Lozenges, suckers and hard candies infused with cannabis can have much the same effect as tinctures and suspensions given that they are sublingually driven products

For foods like snacks, vegetables, entrees, or desserts the GI tract gradually absorbs cannabinoids over the course of one to two hours. This means that it may take an hour or two to feel the effects, both from a pain relief standpoint, as well as a euphoric one.

Ingested cannabis medicine is processed first by the liver, which converts some cannabinoids, especially, THC to slightly different THC molecules (i.e., delta 9 to hydroxy 11). As well, cannabis delivered by edible requires four to ten times the amount of sublingual or even smoked cannabis in order to achieve the same relief. For these reasons' edibles can present a problem in achieving the required or desired dose level in a consistent fashion, especially for patients new to this therapy.

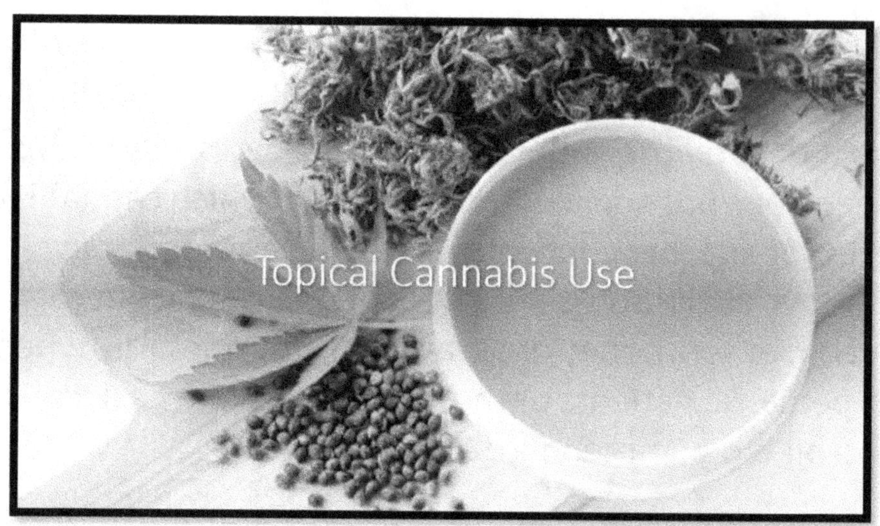

Topical Cannabis Use

Topical applications of cannabis salves, lotions, balms or massage oils will provide the patient with a body effect, primarily noticed as a relaxant, much like a muscle relaxer, but with added bonus of pain relief. Topical applications should be used sparingly until the body affect is known and experienced.

Topicals reduce pain where it occurs, while internal routes increase the brain's resistance to incoming pain signals. Arthritis sufferers are the most common topical cannabis users, although patients have reported rapidly healing third degree burns, experienced relief from eczema, psoriasis, atopic dermatitis, and even cleared poison ivy and poison oak rashes.

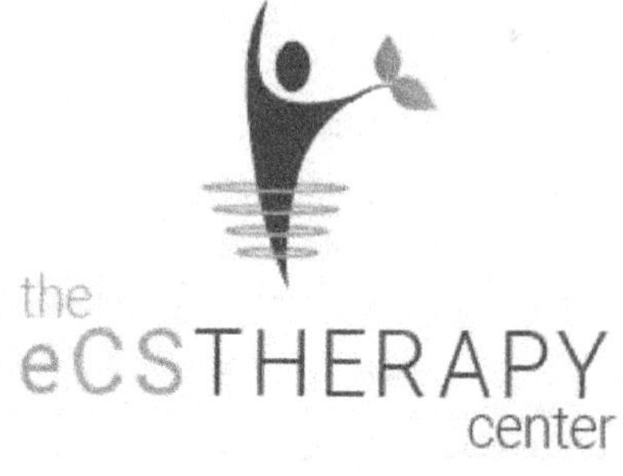

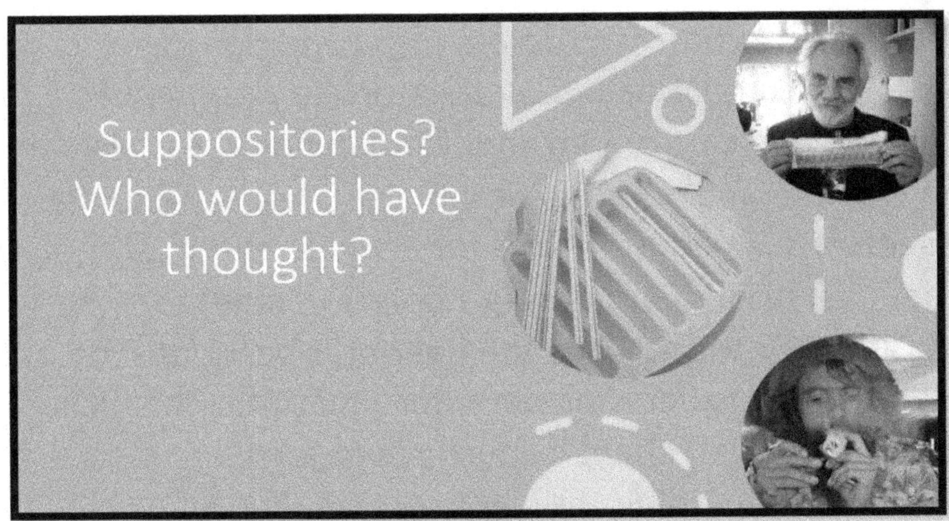

Suppositories

Rectal administrations have an unfair reputation in the U.S. despite the diverse benefits they offer, patients rarely consider them. There are many advantages to a cannabis suppository not afforded by other delivery routes. To start, cannabis may still be administered even if the oral route is impaired, due to vomiting, an injured or broken jaw, swollen or impaired throat, gastro-intestinal difficulties, seizure activity, or other impairment (temporary or permanent) or when oral intake restrictions are in place before and after surgery. Avoiding the GI tract also prevents first-pass metabolism by the stomach and liver, which as mentioned, breaks down many of the cannabinoid components.

Note: Vaginal suppositories will be administered with similar effects. Using suppositories in this manner can provide much relief to issues like endometriosis, adenomyosis, severe menstrual cramps, herpes, and other painful issues.

Note: Though many cannabis patients use suppositories successfully, not everyone will have a positive experience. Uptake for cannabinoids or fats through the colon is known to be less effective than a non-fat or water-soluble drug, so a nano-emulsified cannabis product may have a better uptake potential than FECO, for example.

As the Cannacian® courses progress into condition specific cannabis recommendations and target dosing, remember the biggest difference from an endocannabinoid perspective between children and adults is simply size/weight. Diluting cannabis into a suspension allows for a wide-variety of dosing options: from micro-dosing (only 1 – 2 mg) to macro-dosing (50+ mgs). Since the patient is being dosed with a non-toxic food versus a potentially harmful chemical compound (or several) there is much room for experimentation at finding the right combination of cannabinoids, proper long-term dose, and symptom relief.

Remember earlier we discussed that:

1 gram of Cannabis Oil

=

1 ml of Cannabis Oil

=

1000 mg of Cannabis Oil
(approximately)

To create a Suspension simply Dilute the Cannabis Oil by mixing the following ingredients well:

1 gram of Cannabis Oil

+

2 ounces of Olive Oil (or other oil)

Fill a **1 ml syringe** with *Diluted* Cannabis Oil Suspension:

1 ml of Cannabis Oil Suspension / .25 ml of CO Suspension

=

16 mg of cannabis oil / 4 mg of cannabis oil

Notes

____

____

____

____

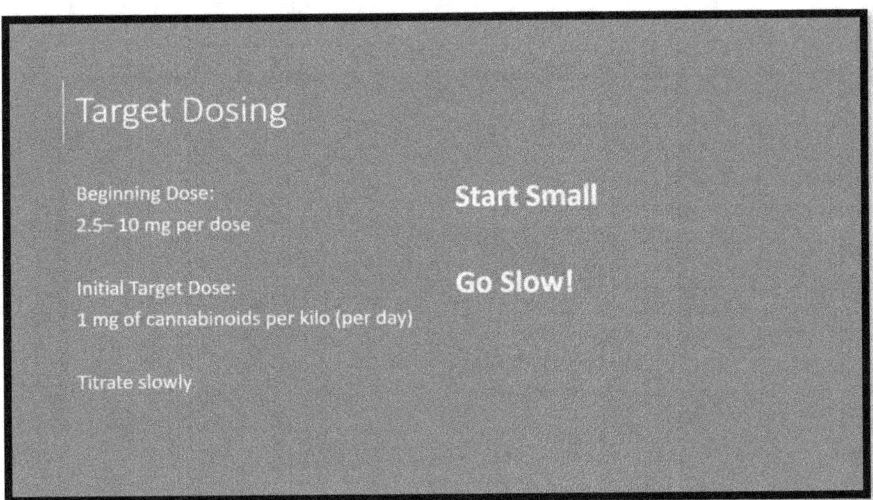

Target dosing is always the same for new patients (or those who have not yet achieved a therapeutic dose of cannabis). Never begin with more than a 5- 10 mg per dose (beginning with only 2.5 mgs for patients who've never used cannabis). Maintain the daily dose at least 3 days before increasing individual doses. Slowly titrate to 1 mg per kilo. Although this is the first target, a majority of people find this dose meets their medical needs regardless of condition they are treating. It may take an adult several weeks or even months to achieve the 1 mg per kilo target (children are typically immediately at the target).

Kilo = 2.2 pounds (lbs)

Daily Cannabis Intake

Mg per Kilo vs Pound

Weight by pound	1/mg per kilo	5/mg per kilo	10/mg per kilo
10	4.5	25	45
20	9	45	91
30	14	68	136
40	18	91	182
50	23	114	227
60	27	136	273
70	32	159	318
80	36	182	364
90	41	205	409
100	45	227	455
110	50	250	500
120	55	273	545
130	59	295	591
140	64	318	636
150	68	341	682
160	73	364	727
170	77	386	773
180	82	409	818
190	86	432	864
200	91	455	909
210	95	477	955
220	100	500	1000

(lbs.) ______ / 2.2 = 1 mg per kilo

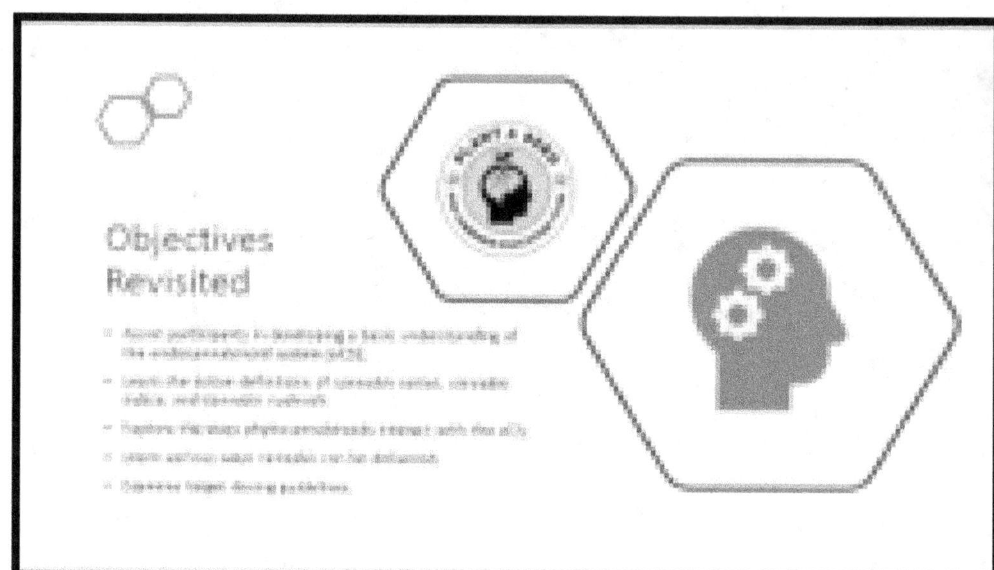

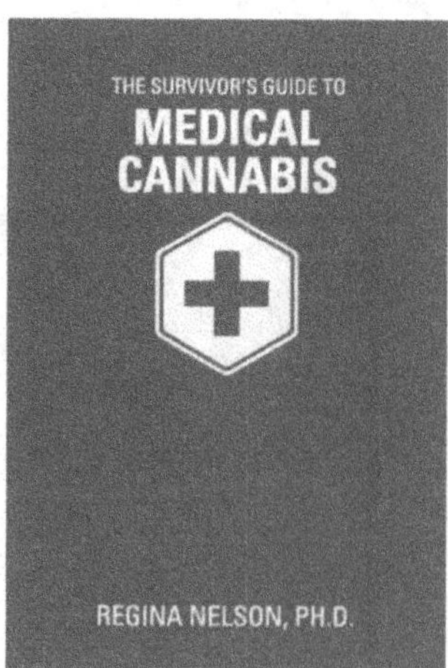

Conclusion

Q & A

Notes

Notes

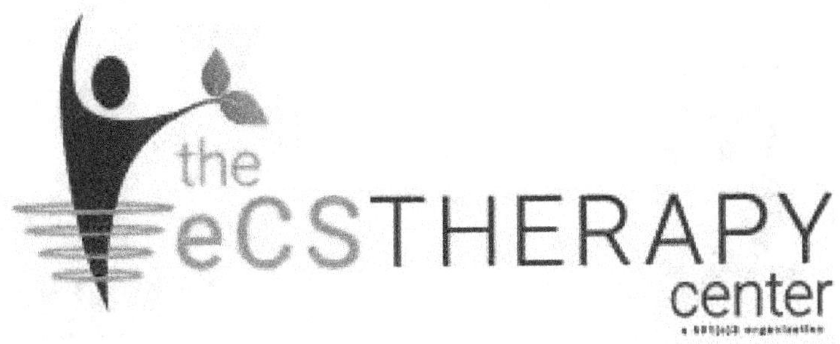
the
eCSTHERAPY
center
a 501(c)3 organization

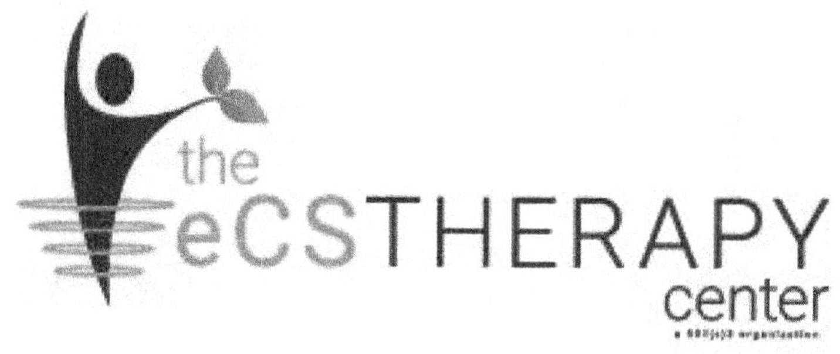

Welcome to
Hemp v. Cannabis
What's the difference?

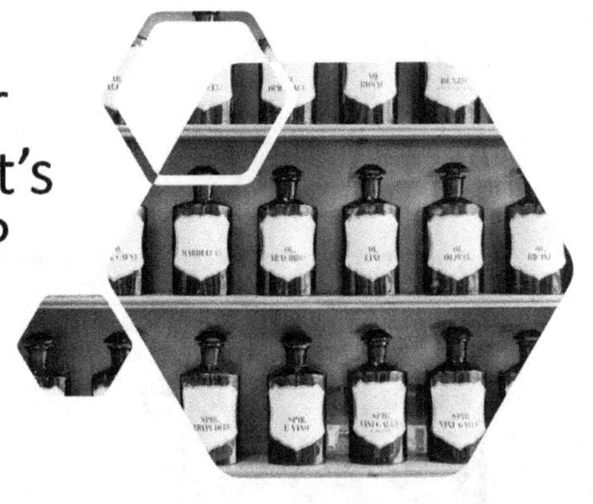

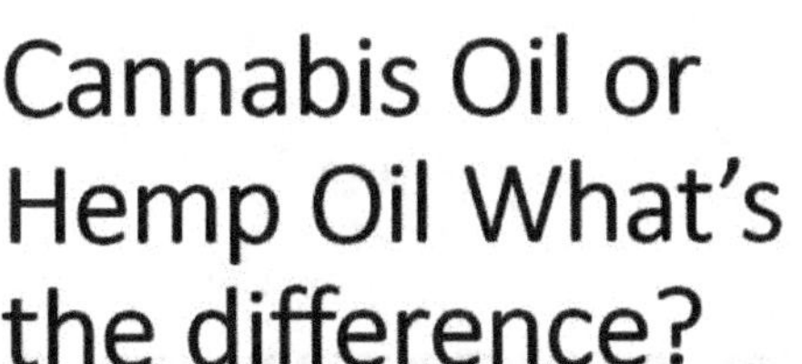

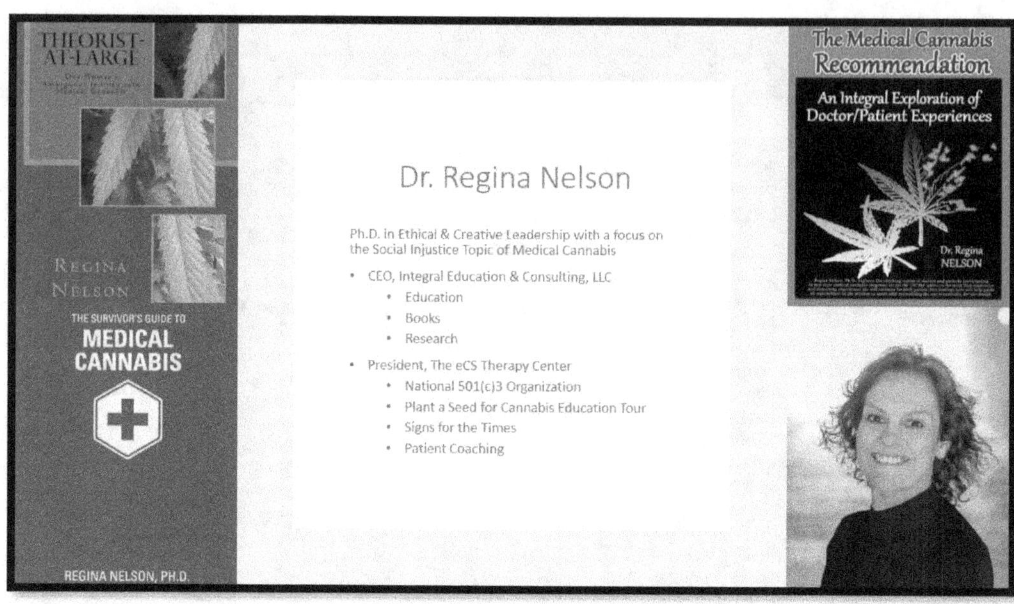

THEORIST-AT-LARGE
REGINA NELSON
THE SURVIVOR'S GUIDE TO
MEDICAL CANNABIS
REGINA NELSON, PH.D.
The Medical Cannabis Recommendation
An Integral Exploration of Doctor/Patient Experiences
Dr. Regina NELSON
Dr. Regina Nelson
Ph.D. in Ethical & Creative Leadership with a focus on the Social Injustice Topic of Medical Cannabis
CEO, Integral Education & Consulting, LLC
Education
Books
Research
President, The eCS Therapy Center
National 501(c)3 Organization
Plant a Seed for Cannabis Education Tour
Signs for the Times
Patient Coaching

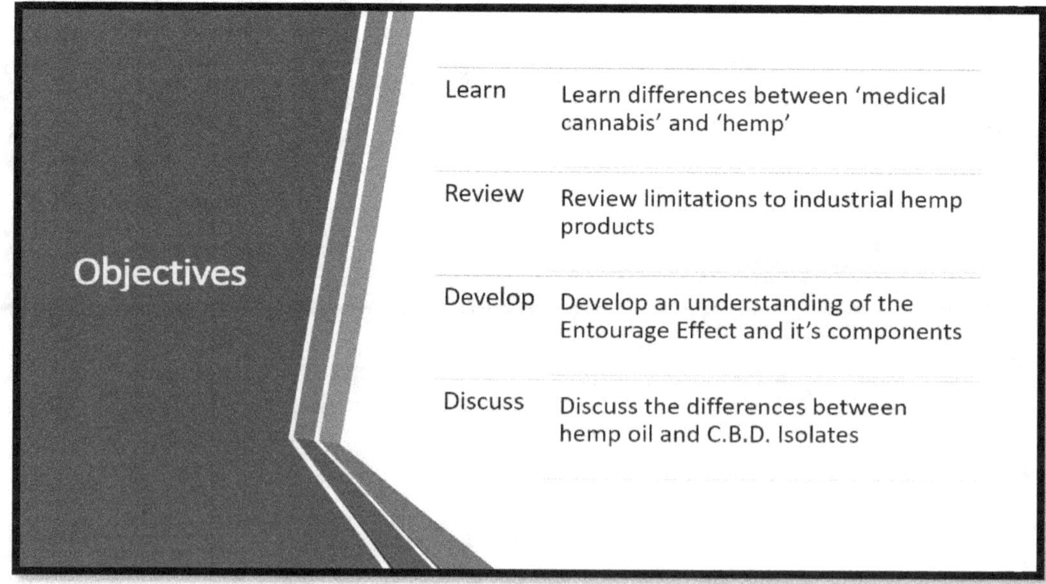

Objectives
Learn   Learn differences between 'medical cannabis' and 'hemp'
Review   Review limitations to industrial hemp products
Develop   Develop an understanding of the Entourage Effect and it's components
Discuss   Discuss the differences between hemp oil and C.B.D. Isolates

From John McPartland's ICRS Presentation

Correct(ed) Vernacular Nomenclature

	INDICA (FORMERLY "SATIVA")	AFGHANICA (FORMERLY "INDICA")	SATIVA (FORMERLY "RUDERALIS")
ORIGINAL PROVENANCE:	India	Central Asia (Afghanistan, Turkestan, Pakistan)	Usually feral or wild C. sativa from Europe, but sometimes of Asian provenance.
MORPHOLOGY:	Relatively tall (ca. ≥1.5 m), laxly branched, with sparsely lanceolate leaflets, and relatively sparse flowering tops.	Relatively short (ca. 0.6-1.5 m), densely branched, with broad leaflets often oblanceolate, and dense flowering tops.	Variable, depending on provenance
PHYSIOLOGY:	Flowering time (seed germination to initiation of reproduction structures under natural conditions) long, 9-14 weeks, no frost tolerance, moderate resin production.	Flowering time short, 7-9 weeks; frost tolerance, high resin production, susceptible to mold	Flowering time relatively short but variable, sometimes autoflowering; moderate frost tolerance, relatively low resin production.
CHEMISTRY:	THC much greater than CBD, uniquely prominent terpenoids: sabinene, α-terpinolene, trans-β-ocimene, trans-β-farnesene, imparting a flowery fragrance	Cannabinoid profile variable (THC greater than or roughly equal to CBD), uniquely prominent terpenoids: camphene, β-myrcene, guaiol, β- and γ-eudesmol, imparting an acrid fragrance	CBD>THC, prominent terpenoids β-caryophyllene, myrcene, imparting a flowery fragrance.
PSYCHOACTIVITY:	"Stimulating."	"Sedating."	Usually lacking.
MEDICAL INDICATIONS:	Lethargic depression, nausea, appetite stimulation, migraine headaches, and chronic pain. Relative contraindications: insomnia, anxiety, and schizophrenia.	Insomnia, anxiety, chronic pain, joint stiffness and inflammation, muscle spasms, tremors (from multiple sclerosis and Parkinson's disease), and epilepsy. Relative contraindications: lethargic depression, somnolence, and schizophrenia.	Chronic pain, joint stiffness and inflammation, epilepsy. Relative contraindications: allergy to cannabis.

REVISED VERNACULAR NOMENCLATURE was proposed by John McPartland at the 2014 meeting of the International Cannabinoid Research Society. His paper, co-authored by Geoffrey Guy, used "DNA barcodes" to determine whether or not *Cannabis indica* and *Cannabis sativa* are separate species. The answer was not. *C. indica* and *C. sativa* are subspecies – separate varieties of one *Cannabis* species. McPartland traced the confusion that prevails today among plant breeders and the pot-loving masses to the 1970s, when a *C. afghanica* plant collected by botanist Richard Evans Schultes was incorrectly identified as *C. indica*.

Cannabis Sativa or Cannabis Ruderalis

The Botany of Cannabis

Botanists that study cannabis and hemp have shared that "we - in the industry" and "we - patients" have our cannabis botany terminology WRONG.

In the industry the widely-held belief is that:
Cannabis Sativa is uplifting and euphoric (and it is, and this is because sativa breed strains contain terpenes like limonene and alpha-pinene which are responsible for the uplifting effects) and sativa plants are thought to be tall and lanky with long, thin finger-like tips.

Cannabis Indica is mellow and relaxing (and it is, and this is because indica-dominant plants contain myrcene, a terpene known for its relaxant side-effects) and these plants are thought to be short or bushy with short, fat finger-like tips.

Cannabis Ruderalis is hemp.

It is true that most cannabis we come into contact with is a hybrid of two or more of these combinations. However, Durban Poison a popular 'true land race sativa' is classified as *cannabis indica* in botany terms because of its high THC content. How confusing is this for current cannabis consumers? Well it gets more confusing...

OLD TERM : NEW TERM   DEFINED AS:
Sativa   Indica   — High THC
Indica   Afghanica —   More Balanced THC:CBD Ratio
Ruderalis   Sativa   — Industrial Use / Very Low THC:CBD

As you can see this is a terminology mess, but it is important to keep in mind that as culture shifts language changes, at some point 'we' must come to communicate in the same terms as scientists. But, I can't say when or how that will happen.

Notes

____

____

____

____

____

____

____

____

____

The Science of
Cannabidiol
(C.B.D.)

$C_{21}H_{30}O_2$

- Cancer
- Heart disease
- Addiction
- Depression
- Seizure disorders (some)
- Stress relief
- Digestive System issues
- MORE....

The Science of C.B.D.

Scientists are beginning to understand the specific pharmacological mechanisms underlying CBD's potential as a treatment for cancer, heart disease, addiction, depression and numerous other health disorders. Cannabidiol is a complex compound that produces many effects through multiple molecular pathways in the body. CBD can penetrate cell membrane and bind to receptors which regulate gene expression and mitochondrial activity. In other words, they have stem cell properties—particularly CBD-A shows this promise, which is quite exciting.

Cannabinoid isolates are NOT the same as whole plant cannabis options that contain other cannabis compounds. Further, CBD isolates (which are very prevalent) behave differently in the body than do whole plant therapies, leaving many consumers disappointed in CBD products and their therapeutic results.

I suggest a full spectrum hemp oil product for those determining if CBD may meet their health needs.

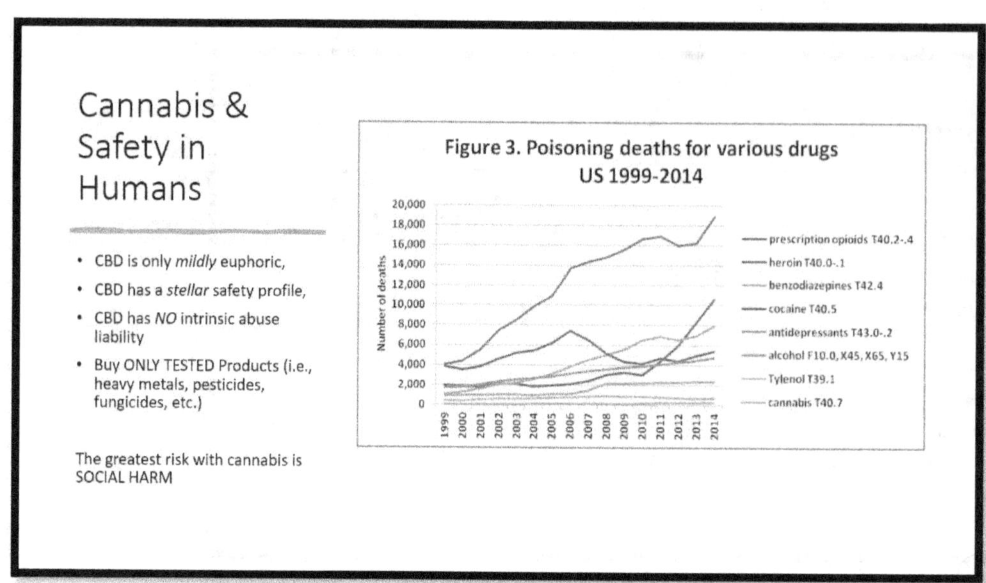

Despite the fact that significant scientific evidence shows that cannabis is non-toxic, free of harmful side-effects, is neurogenerative, neuroprotective, and every human being has an endocannabinoid system, we cannot lose sight of the fact that *cannabis sativa* remains a Schedule One drug, which means it is classified as being highly dangerous, highly addictive and non-medicinal.

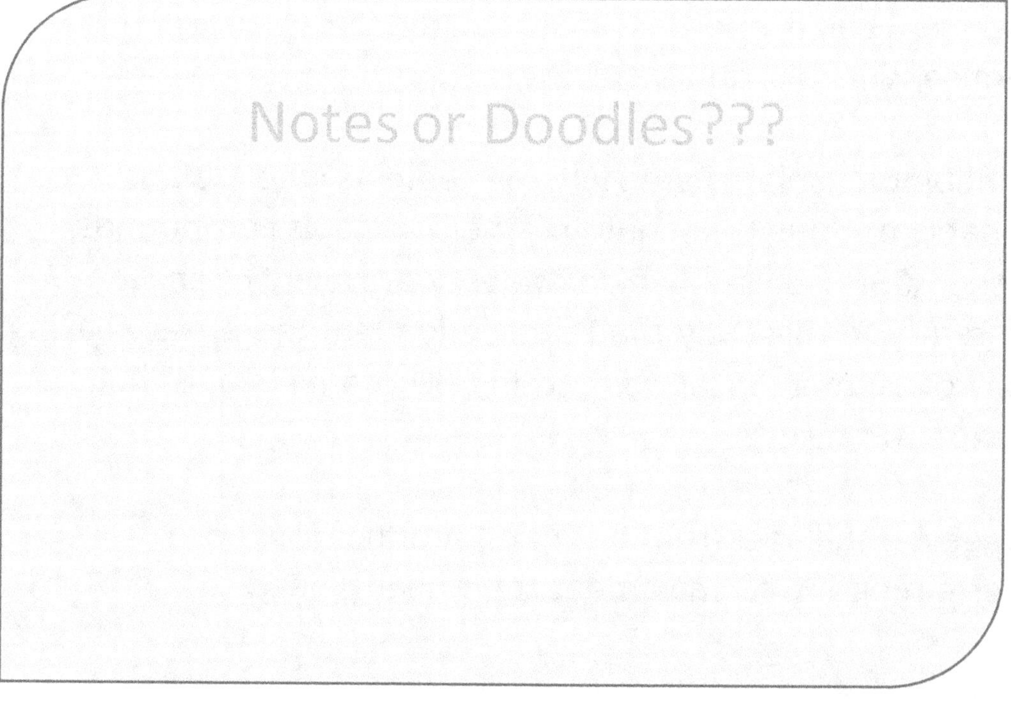

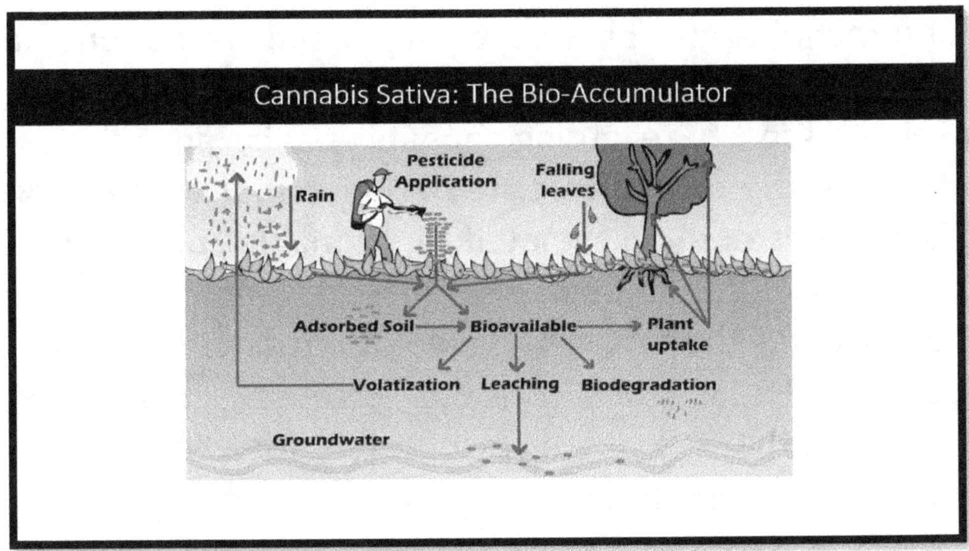

Cannabis: A Bio-Accumulative Plant

A huge amount of industrial hemp is required to extract a small amount of CBD. This raises the risk of contaminants as hemp is a "bio-accumulator"—meaning the plant naturally draws toxins from the soil.

In short, pesticides and other chemicals used on industrial and even agricultural food crops, get absorbed by plants that are bio-accumulators. The plants ingest the pesticides and other chemicals and unless the bio-accumulative plant is destroyed or used for industrial purposes, the 'icides' get passed up the food chain.

Types of pesticides: Herbicides (kill plants) Insecticides (kill insects) Fungicides (kill fungus) and Bactericides (kill bacteria)

TERPENES

Terpenes or terpenoids give plants their smell and are not unique to the cannabis plant. However, Dr. Ethan Russo (2019) made a very interesting discovery regarding cannabis strains and terpenes. In short, **the only difference between indica and sativa strains as known currently in the medical cannabis community is one thing; a certain terpene, *myrcene*.** Russo's research is among the first that validates the medicinal value of terpenes. As well, it demonstrates that THC is THC, CBD is CBD, etcetera—it is instead, the terpene profile that is primarily responsible for differing effects between cannabis strains.

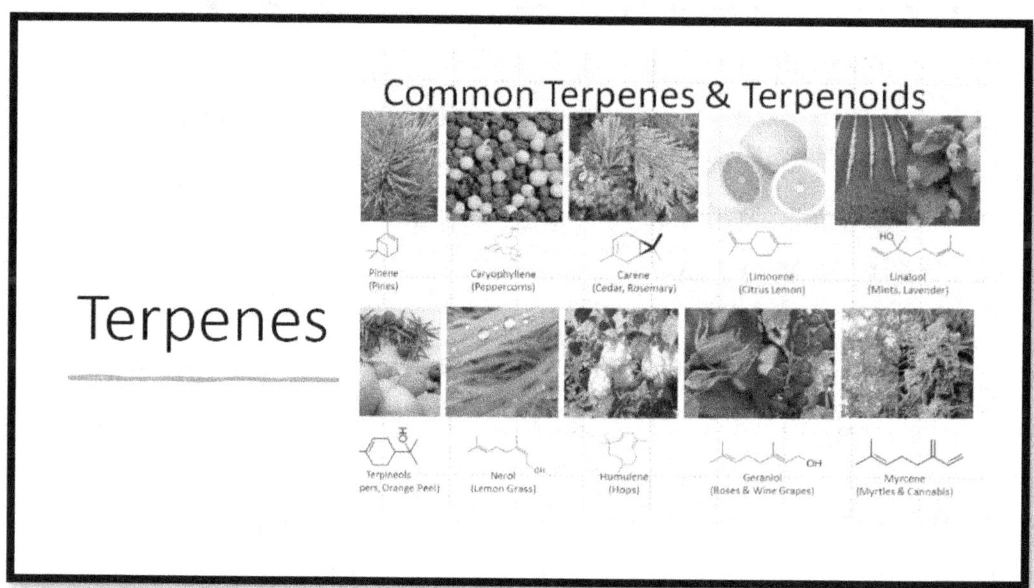

The Survivor's Guide to Medical Cannabis dives deeper into this topic.

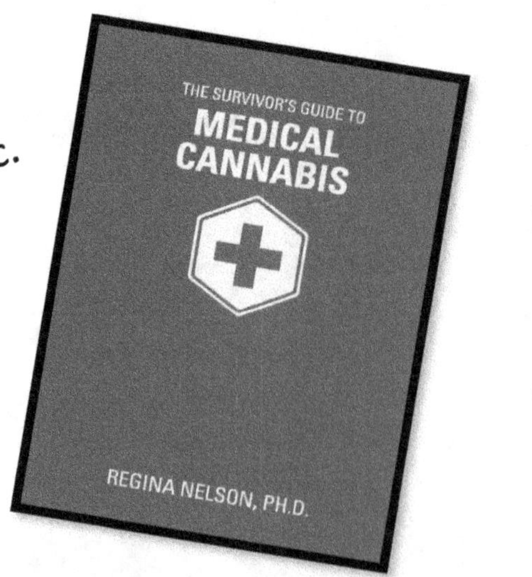

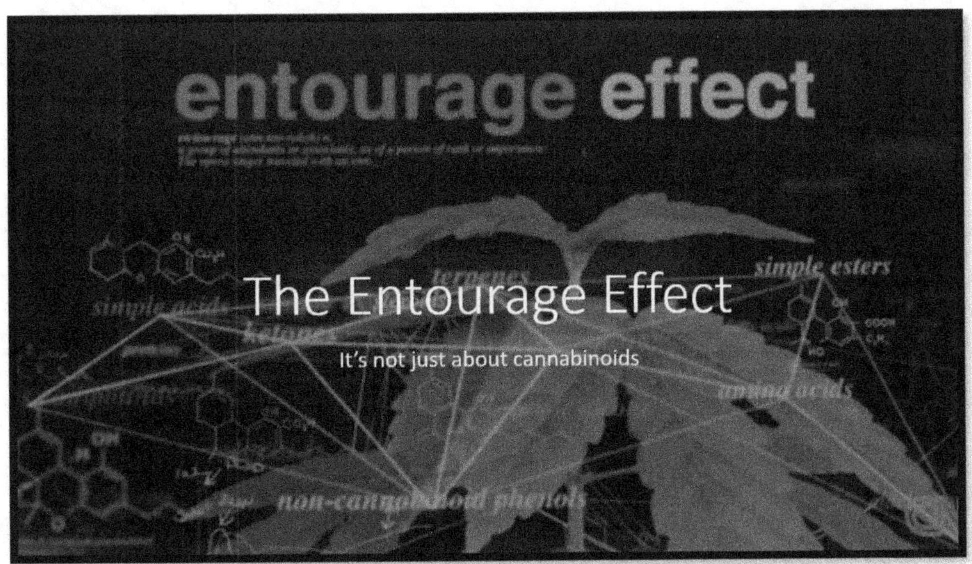

The Entourage Effect

There is well documented evidence of the entourage effect—isolates and hemp derivatives are often missing the key entourage components: CBG, CBC, minor cannabinoids, terpenes, flavonoids…and yes, even THC.

Notes

____

____

____

____

____

____

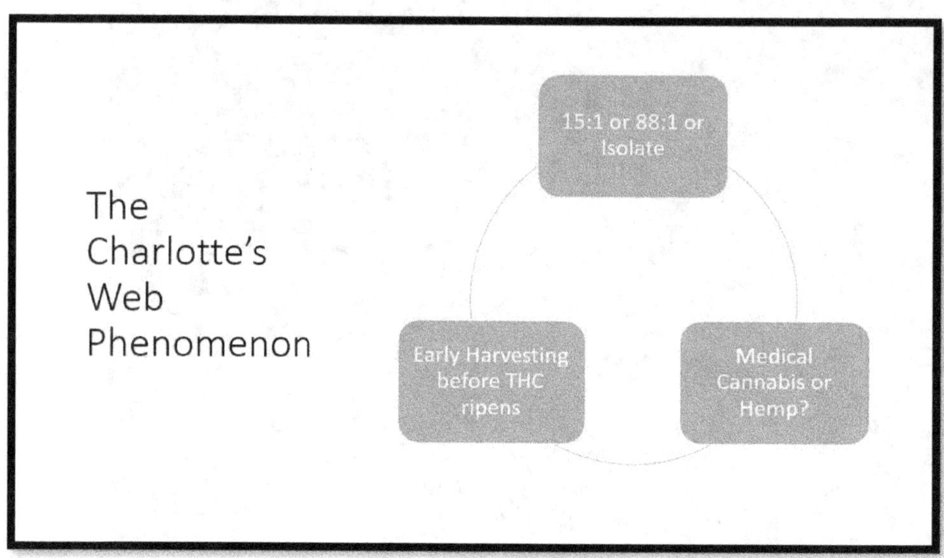

In *The Survivor's Guide to Medical Cannabis*, I explain that much media attention has been given to one particular CBD-rich strain, Charlotte's Web—and yet, it is certainly not the only or perhaps even the best strain for those seeking CBD-rich therapies. For example, Charlotte's Web, now CW, has become branded, and as with most brands, it's been modified significantly from its original label (I.e., formula). Today's this brand's Hemp Oil (88:1) is not the same as the Cannabis Oil (15: 1 - 22:1), which was given attention on CNN's *Weed* Special by Dr. Sanjay Gupta in 2013. This is not a bad thing, it's just something most people don't recognize because of the way it was talked about when it was a 15 – 22:1 ratio of medical cannabis instead of true hemp oil.

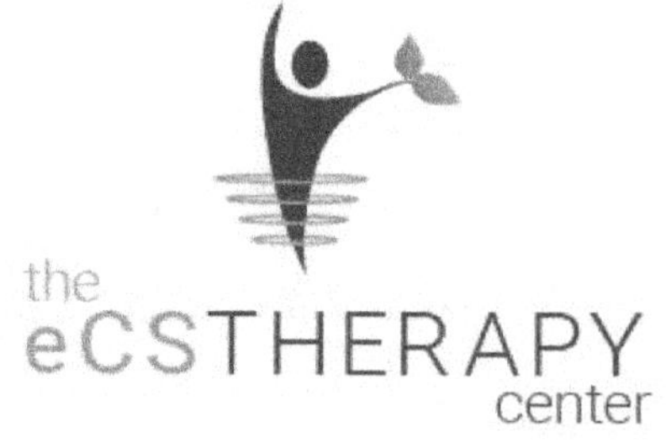

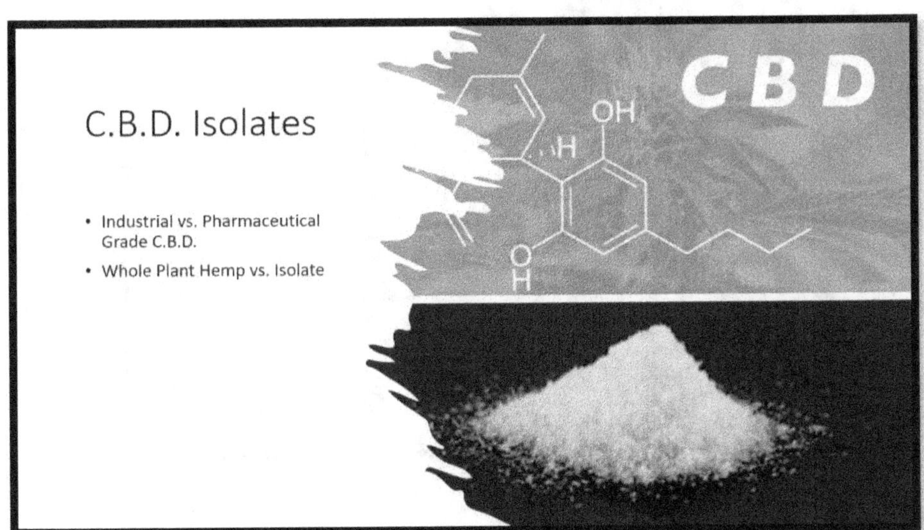

C.B.D. Isolates

The pharmaceutical development of *synthetic* cannabinoid compounds is based upon controlled experimentation with molecular isolates in keeping with the assumption that sick people benefit most from predictable, reproducible medicine that never varies. While pharmaceutical isolates can facilitate precision dosage and confidence in the chemical make-up of a drug, these isolated cannabinoids, especially synthetic ones, do not react the same within the body as whole plant extracts.

Note: A 2016 study by Italian researchers found that a whole plant CBD-rich oil extract "attenuated inflammation and hypermotility" (i.e., diarrhea) in an animal model of colitis, whereas "pure CBD did not ameliorate colitis" symptoms. In the researchers' words, "These findings sustain the rationale of combining CBD with other cannabis constituents (i.e., the entourage effect is real) and support the clinical development of CBD [as a] *botanical* drug substance for irritable bowel disease treatment."

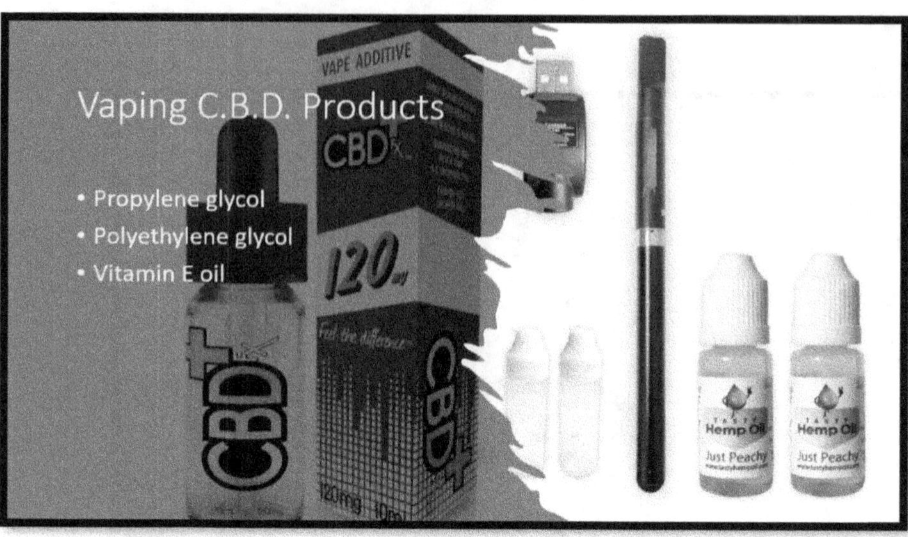

Vaping C.B.D.

If vaping products were regulated to prohibit the use of toxic thinning agents and flavoring additives, then they'd be safe— until that time unless the product is hemp oil or cannabis oil derived, I don't recommend their use. Several additives (propylene glycol and polyethylene glycol, for example) that are commonly found in CBD vape cartridges become toxic when heated and inhaled.

Also keep in mind, that most flavoring additives have not been safety tested for inhalation; even though some are known to be highly toxic when combusted. Vape industry insiders are well aware that the flavoring and other additives are connected to popcorn lung issues.

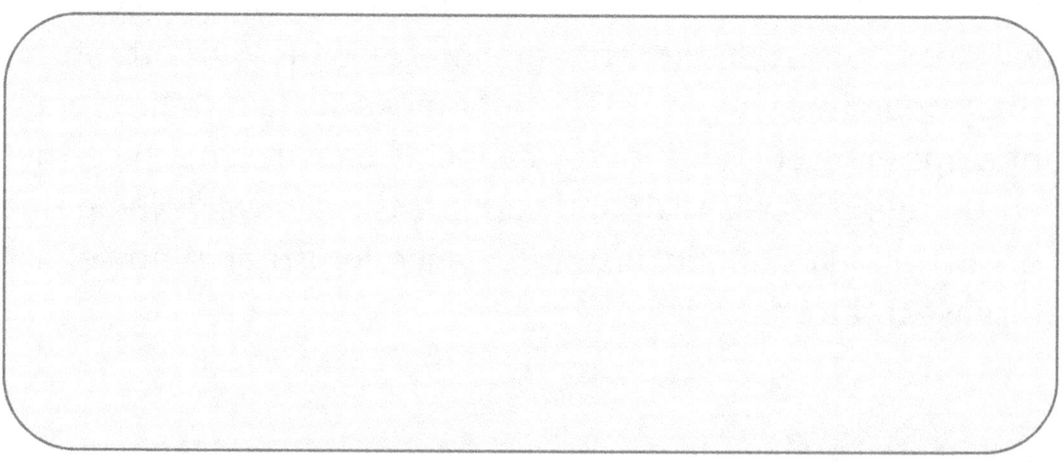

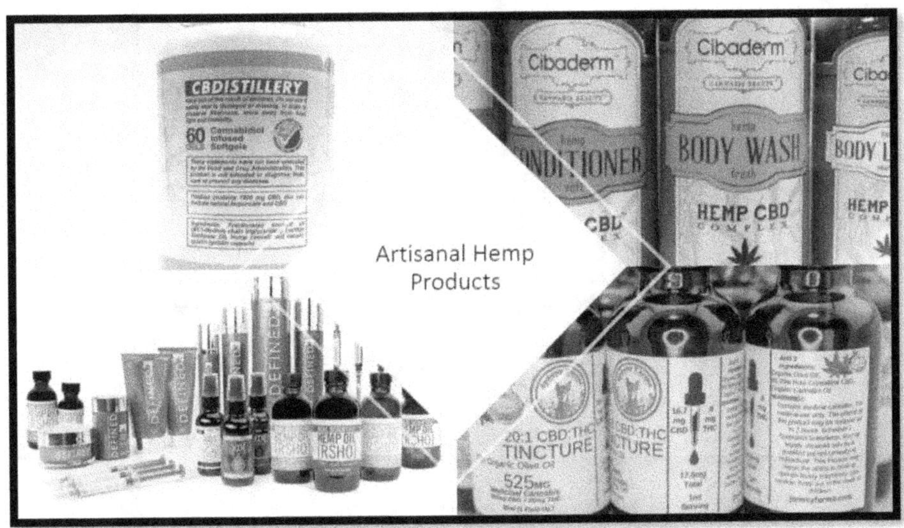

Artisanal Hemp Products

The business of developing hemp products is burgeoning, but the biggest question comes with each and every new product, what's this made of? Is it a natural hemp oil extraction? Is it a tainted Chinese industrial hemp import? Is this pharmaceutical grade CBD isolate? What is in it?

Notes

____

____

____

____

____

____

____

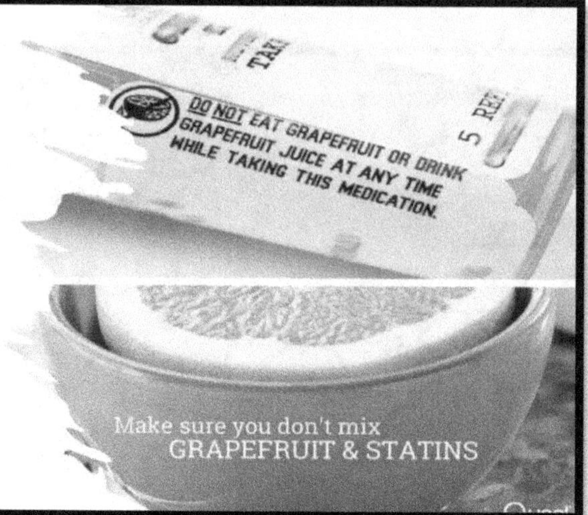

Hemp Oil vs. C.B.D. Isolates

(Note: For more information on CBD Isolates v. Hemp Oil visit www.projectcbd.org operated by Martin Lee).

A recent study states "Problematic drug interactions are much more likely with high doses of single-molecule CBD (i.e., CBD isolate), **which can inhibit the metabolism of 60 percent of marketed pharmaceuticals.**"

IF a pharmaceutical label warns that the drug should not be taken with grapefruit or grapefruit juice, one should not engage in therapy with a CBD isolate.

This warning also applies to pregnant women as large doses of CBD isolate may be related to placenta abruption problems.

BUT- keep in mind - we do not see these drug interaction as frequently with hemp oil products.

Pharmaceutical Grade Isolates are NOT Whole Plant Products

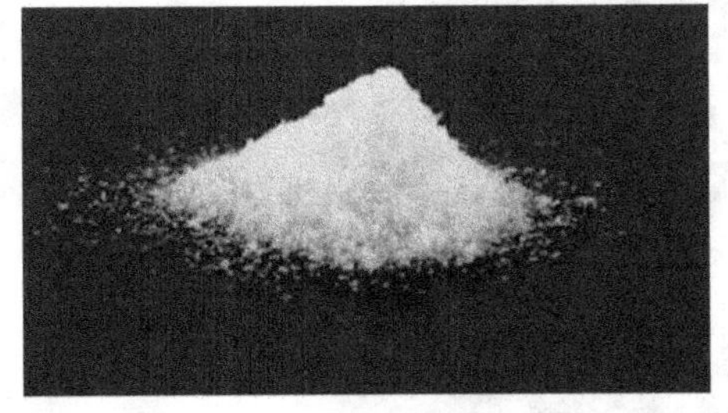 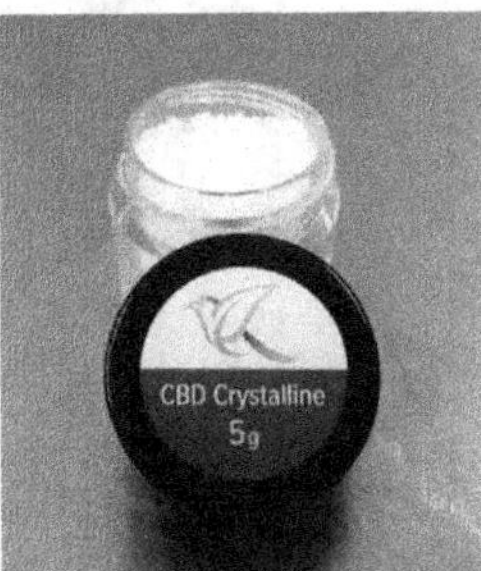

Pharmaceutical grade CBD is but one isolate cannabinoid,(it is important, but it works best in unison with other compounds from the cannabis plant).

With isolates, even safe ones:
There is NO Entourage Effect
It may be of Questionable Quality
Is it an industrial or pharmaceutical grade isolate? Do you know?

How does the patient plan to deliver the isolate?
Smoking?
Vaporizing?
Edibles?
Topical application?
Or another way?

Unless the isolate is used
to boost a whole plant
Product, I avoid them.

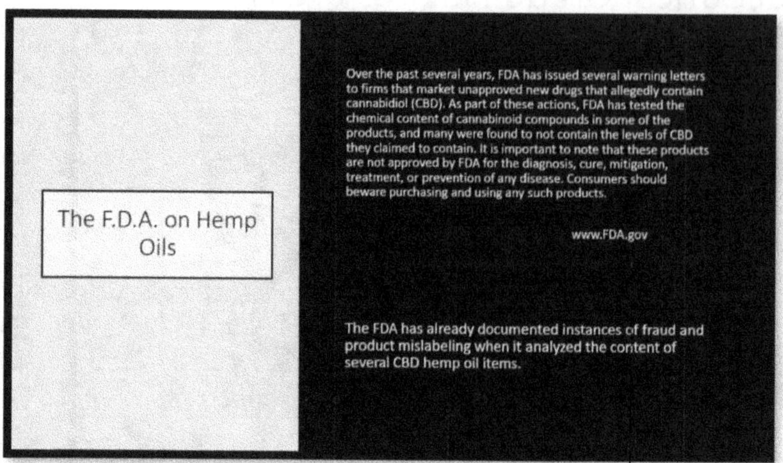

Food & Drug Administration Warnings on CBD

Reading the labels of CBD products can be quite confusing. Even the F.D.A. (U.S. Food and Drug Administration) has weighed in on the quality (or lack thereof) in these types of products. If you visit their website fda.gov you will find they have accumulated a long list of products claiming to be "CBD products" that either contained no CBD or other cannabinoids and/or were contaminated by heavy metals or pesticides.

Notes

____

____

____

____

____

____

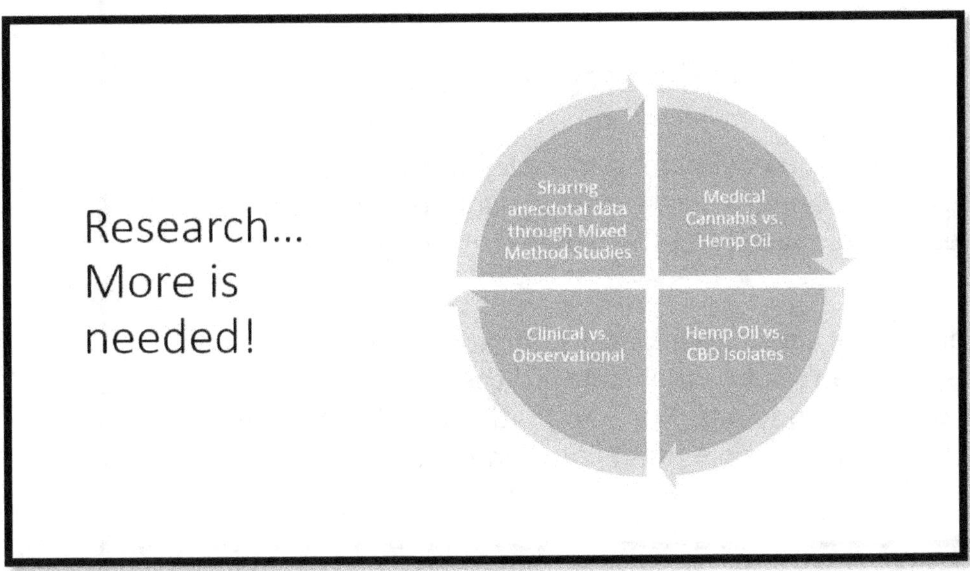

Though we are starting to see more research dedicated to CBD, it is important that we fast track clinical studies designed to compare the efficacy of CBD isolates and whole plant CBD-rich extracts because companies are marketing and people are using them now.

Notes

____

____

____

____

____

____

Hope for the Future

Pure CBD is a molecule, not a miracle, and it doesn't work for everyone. No-THC and low-THC cannabis oil products represent a small slice of the cannabis therapy spectrum.

Patients of all ages and economic means should have access to a range of cannabis-based therapeutic options with different concentrations and ratios of CBD and THC, along with other whole plant components.

Five years ago, finding CBD rich products was next to impossible, now retail stores specializing in CBD have sprung up across the globe. In the quickly changing mainstream market product lines now feature hemp oil extracts and CBD supplements. And, in the U.S. 37 states now support the medical use of cannabis in some legislated fashion—and an ever-growing number of states are also implementing adult use regulations; plus, the U.S. Government has finally approved a Farm Bill that supports CBD cultivated from hemp. I thought by 2022, we would be celebrating "federal legalization" and the removal of cannabis from the Schedule of Controlled Substances—but sadly, it has not yet occurred.

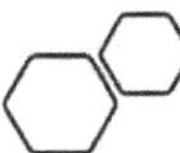

Objectives Revisited

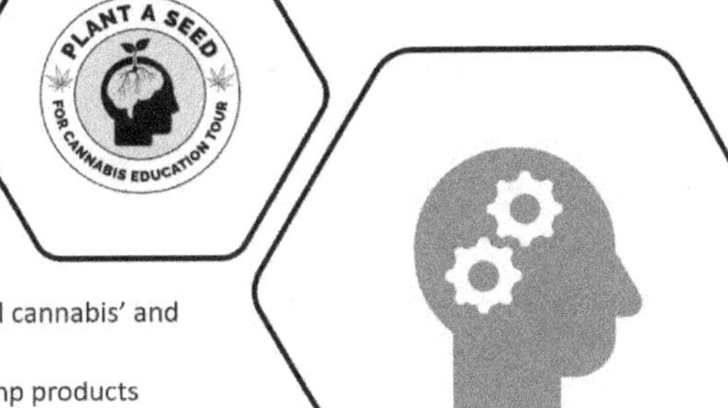

- Learn differences between 'medical cannabis' and 'hemp'
- Review limitations to industrial hemp products
- Develop an understanding of the Entourage Effect and it's components
- Discuss the differences between hemp oil and C.B.D. Isolates

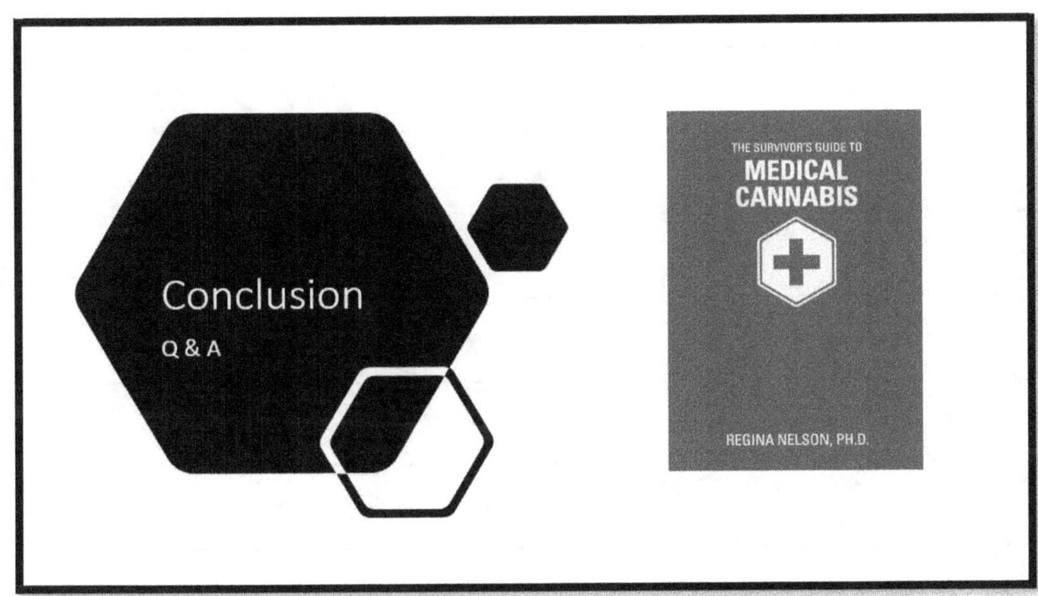

Notes

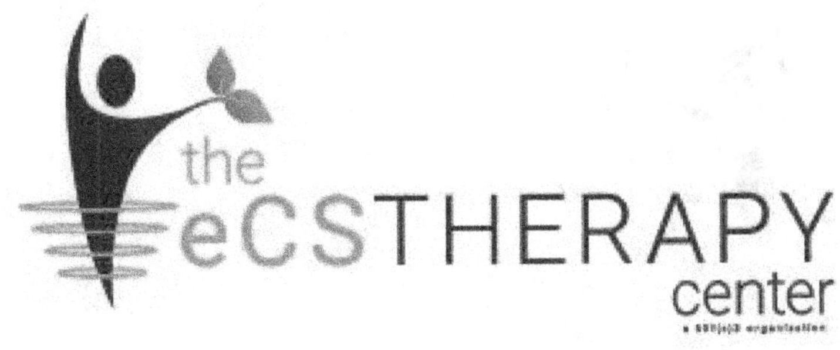

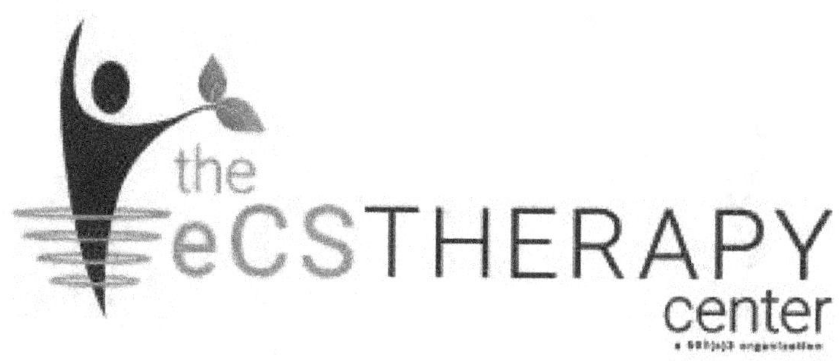

Welcome to
Targeted Dosing Strategies

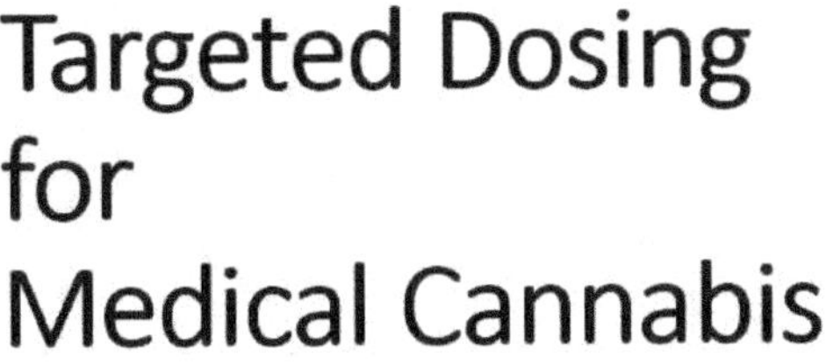

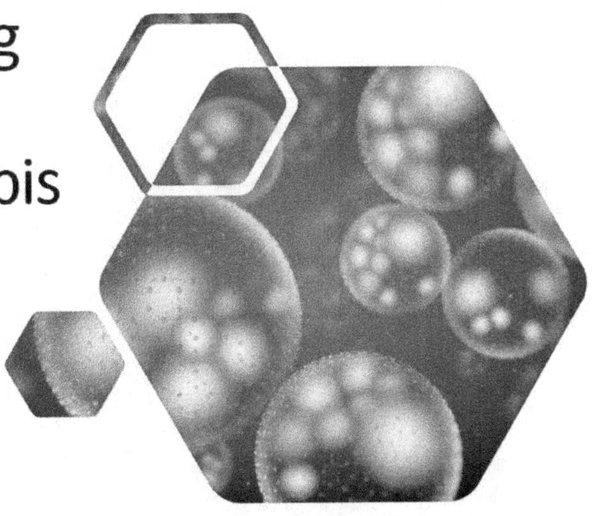

Objectives

Learn | Learn therapeutic dosing targets established in scientific research

Examine | Examine targeted dosing guidelines for patients using medical cannabis therapeutically

Discover | Discover the differences between whole plant cannabis products and cannabinoid isolate products

Understand | Understand how patients can safely and comfortably titrate cannabis medicines

Notes

____

____

____

____

____

____

____

____

____

What's a Therapeutic Dose of Cannabis?

Science
- 1 mg per kilo THC

Animal Studies
- THC vs. CBD 1 mg – 20 mg per kilo
- Condition Specific Targets
  - Pain 1 – 5 mg per kilo
  - Cancer 10 – 20 mg per kilo

Patients Report
- 1-mg of Cannabinoids per Kilo of weight
- 5 – 10 mg per dose to start, with slow and steady titration to 1 mg per kilo daily dose
- Condition Specific Reports

What is a Therapeutic Dose of Cannabis?

Scientists use the guideline of 1 mg per kilo as the minimum therapeutic dose of THC —a singular cannabinoid—in animal studies.

As I have observed patients and have written about in *The Survivor's Guide to Medical Cannabis* if we instead use 1 mg per kilo as the target, but instead of isolating one cannabinoid, we utilize 'cannabinoids' as the 1 mg per kilo target, most patients will find relief early in medical cannabis therapy.

In fact, in my observation, ***1 mg per kilo of cannabinoids*** a day seems to even be ideal long-term daily dose for more than half of the patients who come to use cannabis medicinally. Those who are taking less may feel some relief, but they haven't hit the 'sweet spot.' Once stabilized at the target dose of 1 mg per kilo for a week or more, patients will decide for themselves if more is needed.

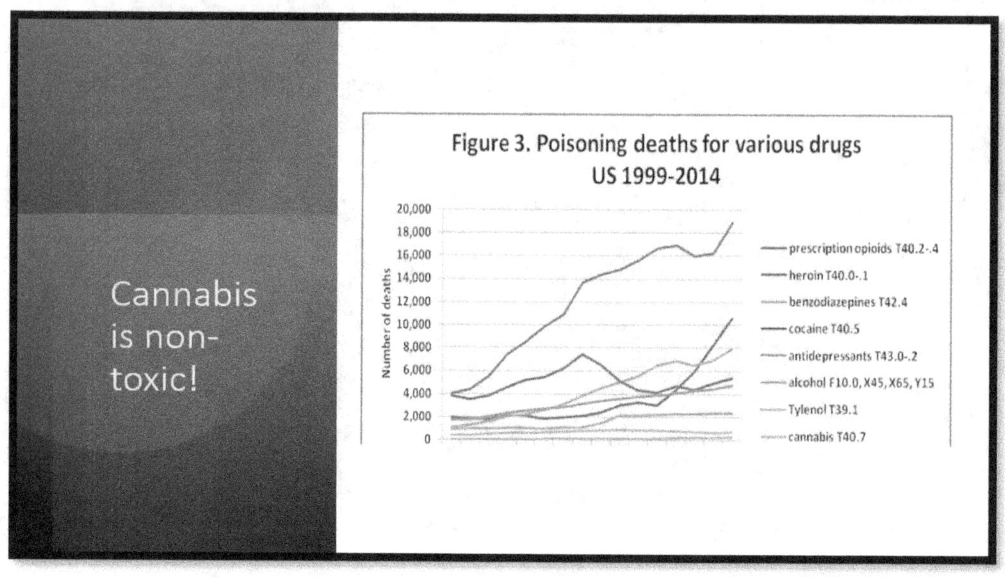

Just a quick reminder that cannabis is non-toxic, and while an over-dose of cannabis may create an uncomfortable experience, it will not lead to death.

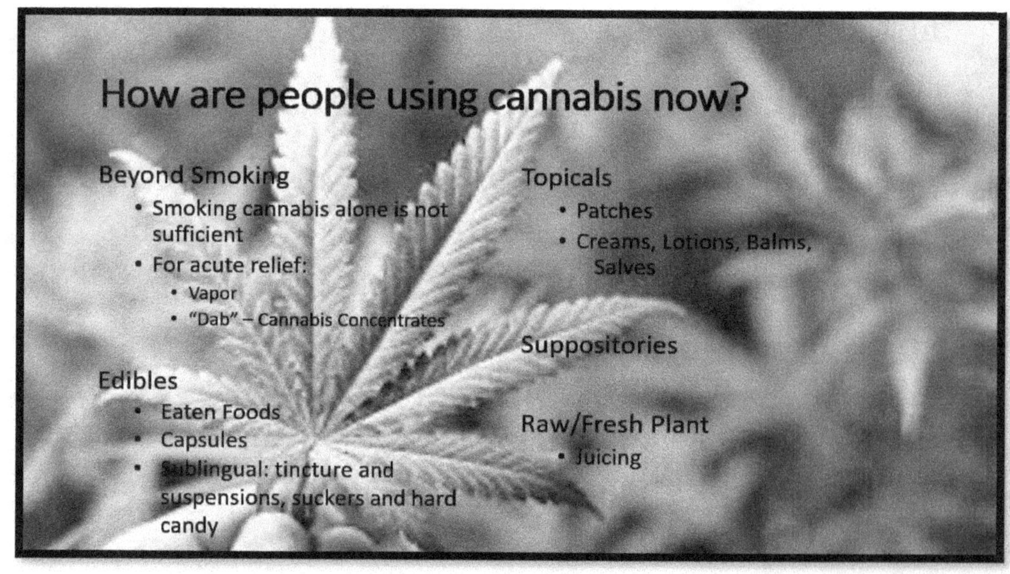

Smoke/Vapor

No one can reach a minimum therapeutic dose of cannabinoids or 1 mg per kilo of cannabis daily by smoking cannabis alone. It is vital that the patient also consumes a cannabis oil regimen or edible foods. That said, smoking is not harmful. For many patients, myself included, smoking cannabis provides relief fast and reliable relief for symptoms like nausea, vomiting, pain, etc. In fact, many pain patients, use 'dabbing' as a means to withdraw from opiates, so smoking and/or vaporizing really should not be discounted as it can be part of a successful cannabis therapy plan.

Edibles

Foods infused with cannabis are excellent for dosing, but they're very different from smoking or tinctures in that they must pass through our digestive system before having effect on symptoms. For foods like snacks, vegetables, entrees, or desserts, the GI tract gradually absorbs cannabinoids over the course of one to two hours. This means that it may take an hour or two to feel the effects; both from a pain relief standpoint, as well as a euphoric one.

Topical

Topical applications of cannabis salves, lotions, balms or massage oils will provide the patient with a body effect, primarily noticed as a relaxant, much like a muscle relaxer, but with an added bonuses of pain relief and ability to function. Patients should use topical
applications sparingly, until the body affect is known and experienced.

Suppositories

There are many advantages to a cannabis suppository not afforded by other delivery routes, even though we don't have enough data to say whether or not this is an effective administration route for large doses of cannabis delivered in an oil-based form. (Note: This may be a great place for nano-emulsification technology).

Raw/Fresh Cannabis Plant

Juicing garden-fresh cannabis is the only ingestion method I've found to be truly non-psychoactive. However, nearly 100% of patients' state that ingesting cannabis juice increases energy, decreases pain, and brings other immediate and long-term benefits. None describe euphoria as a side- effect. Until recently (2018), scientists were befuddled by reports from patient's finding relief with cannabis juice. However, scientists have now demonstrated that THCa, CBDa, and other cannabinoids in their precursor or acid form have significant health benefits that must be considered.

The truth is that if we all consumed cannabis in this manner, just as many people now consume wheatgrass juice or fresh vegetable juices, our society would suffer from less illnesses. As well, our propensity toward the euphoric effects of cannabis would be lessened-- by increasing amounts of cannabinoids circulating through our systems and stored in our bodies the effects even of smoked cannabis would be diminished.

Whole Plant Cannabis vs Cannabis Isolates

Cannabinoid plant chemistry is far more complex than that of any singular cannabinoid of interest—when delivered in a whole plant option, cannabis can be far more effective than when delivered by a cannabinoid isolate. In fact, different effects and symptom relief may be experienced due to a change in cannabinoid or even a terpene profile.

Whole Plant vs Isolates
Where's the *Entourage Effect?*
CBD
Supplement Facts

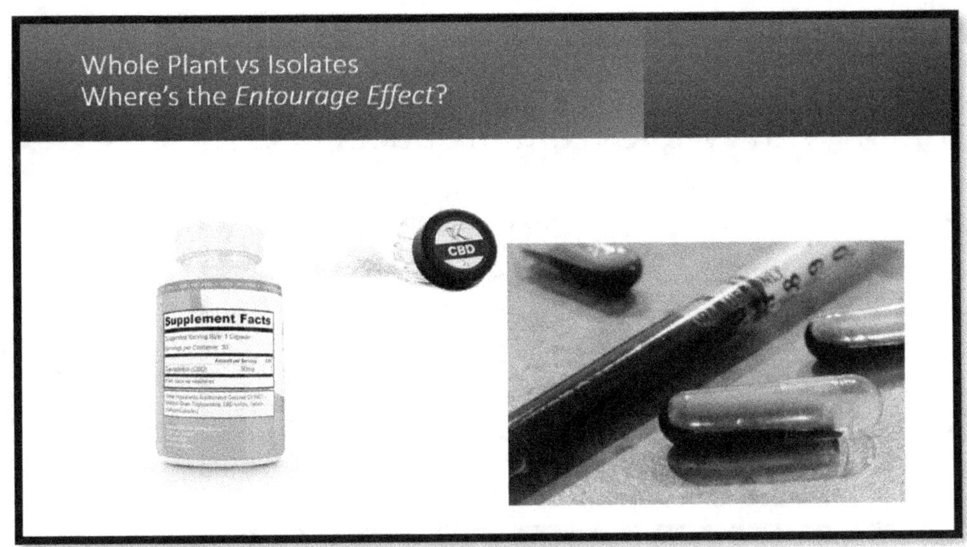

Notes

____

____

____

____

____

____

____

____

____

Titration with Whole Plant Products

Micro-dosing Strategies
- THC-sensitive individuals
- Supplement CBD regiments
- Short-term success

- Begins with 1 – 2mg nighttime dose
- 1 – 2mg starting dose, 4 – 6 x day
- Wait two weeks before increasing the dose

Common Patient Dosing
- One 5 -10mg nighttime dose
- 5 – 10mg starting dose, 4 x day
- Continuous patient assessment of symptoms and side-effects
- Every 3 – 4 days, at least once per week, increase each daily dose by 5 – 10mg
- Bulk up nighttime dose by doubling every 3 – 4 days
- Wait two weeks after reaching Target Dose of 1-mg of cannabinoids per kilo of weight before increasing dose

Titration with Whole Plant Products

Currently there are two dosing theories in the cannabis world: micro-dosing strategies and common patient dosing.

Micro-Dosing

THC sensitive people (or the caregiver of one) need to know that even if the patient has THC-sensitivity, cannabis therapy may still be appropriate. In this case, micro-dosing may be a better option if the patient is using medical cannabis products. It will also help to try low THC options and avoid smoking cannabis.

Microdosing uses 1 - 2.5mg per dose; at least four (4) doses should be given in a day, but more may be provided more often.

Ideally, the patient will take four (4) doses each day: morning, early afternoon, early evening, and bed time. This allows cannabinoids to stay active in the patient's system, as well a storage of cannabinoids will develop in their fat cells (the reason people fail drug tests).

Common Cannabis Patient Dosing

For patients new to cannabis therapy, it is always wise to take the first dose of cannabis at night, regardless of delivery method—that way if the euphoric side-effects are too much the patient can sleep through much of it.

The first dose of cannabis should not exceed 10 mg—for most people, especially those not currently using cannabis, a 5 mg dose is best. This is particularly true if the patient has any fear of the euphoric side-effects.

Ideally, the patient will take four (4) doses each day: morning, early afternoon, early evening, and bed time. More doses may be given each day, but less is not recommended.

In a perfect world, the patient will document their symptoms and side-effects so that others (Cannacians, caregivers, spouses, parents, etc.) can help them understand how the cannabis is working.

Once per week—or as soon as every 3 -4 days—a patient can increase their individual daily doses by 5 – 10 mgs until they reach the 1 mg per kilo target.

The patient should maintain the target dose for about a several weeks before assessing how well cannabis therapy is working for them. A large percentage, perhaps as many as 80 – 90% of people, find sufficient relief at this initial target dose of 1 mg per kilo.

For patients who are trying to titrate up quickly (i.e., cancer patients), increasing the dose at night (much like beginning with a nighttime dose) will help determine if the side-effects will become 'too much' at the increased level.

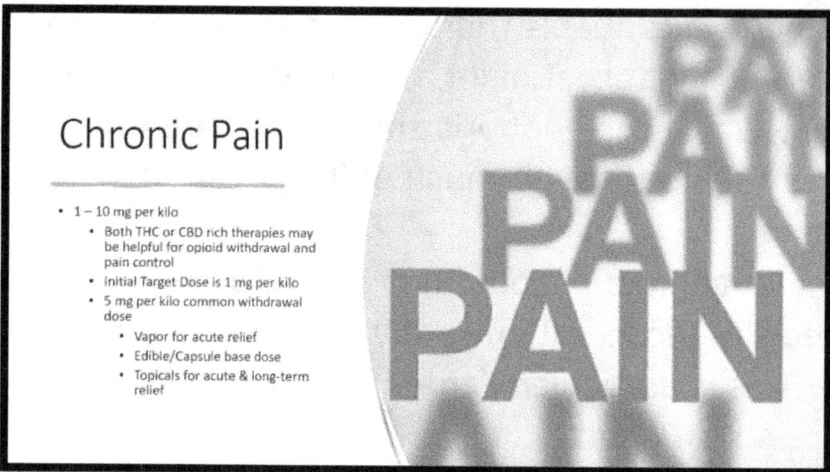

Chronic Pain

Thousands of patients (and several research studies) have described how cannabis treats pain not as a pain-killer, but as a pain-distancer -- removing the patient from the pain, making it more bearable, and allowing them to function despite pain. In fact, chronic pain issues are the #1 reason people seek medical cannabis treatment.

For patients with chronic pain issues it is suggested that they layer cannabis therapies—meaning they should use cannabis in a variety of different ways for maximum relief. For example, a consistent dose of indica-dominant cannabis oil in the 1 - 5 mg per kilo range each day may reduce pain symptoms considerably regardless of the condition or injury contributing to the pain. The addition of topical products on a regular basis, and smoking/ vaporizing cannabis when symptoms are most acute (i.e., patient has a flare), will also provide a great deal of relief.

For those new to cannabis therapy, beginning with a combination of tincture/ suspension or an edible at a very low dose taken several times a day, a topical salve applied several times per day, and vaporizing if the pain is acute will provide maximum relief.

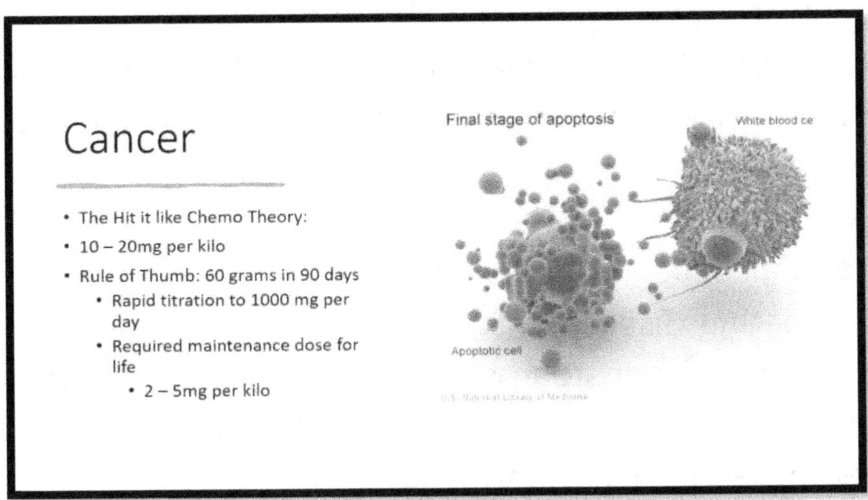

Cancer

Cancer of all types is often caused by imbalances within the body. Frequently cancers are caused for endogenous reasons (system imbalances leading to tumor growth) versus foreign effect (environmental exposures to toxins).

Though oncologists will insist that they recommend cannabis because it helps with the nausea and vomiting associated with chemotherapy (and it does); cannabinoids have repeatedly been shown by researchers to have a positive effect on many types of cancer through a process called apoptosis.

Apoptosis is the process of cellular death and our bodies are constantly in a process of killing off old cells and replacing them with new ones. For example, our skin fully regenerates every four (4) months through an apoptosis process. Sleep is particularly vital to healing in large part because when we sleep our body turns up the programming on apoptosis.

Cancer is basically apoptosis interrupted—cancer cells that should have been killed by the apoptosis process continue to live and breed; eventually a person may have a tumor as a symptom of the cancer. But, a cancerous tumor is just a symptom of apoptosis gone awry in the body. It is also a sign that the endocannabinoid system is having difficulty creating homeostasis. For many any addition of phytocannabinoids can be a helpful supplement to the body's own eCS.

Contrary to popular belief, smoking cannabis does not assist a great deal in treating disease within the body, as therapeutic levels cannot be reached. Instead smoking cannabis provides acute relief of severe symptoms, notably nausea and cachexia caused by chemotherapy treatments, pain, etc.

A cannabis cancer therapy regimen is akin to pulling out the big guns! The patient chooses to engage in a serious cannabis oil regimen and ideally incorporates cannabis juice into the diet, as well as layering any additional therapies that may prove beneficial, such as a topical treatment for symptom and condition treatment. For example, topical applications would be recommended for a patient with skin cancer (i.e., melanoma).

Scientific study and observation suggest a $10 - 20$mg of cannabinoids per kilo of weight target is necessary to truly combat a cancerous situation.

Notes

____

____

____

____

____

In studies cannabis has been shown to improve the efficacy of opioids and narcotics by up to 500%--this means people need fewer opiates or narcotics.

It is also important to remember that CBD has effect at the **P-450 enzyme** (cellular level), meaning that if a patient is prescribed a drug that blocks this enzyme, CBD may adversely affect the pharmaceutical side-effects (i.e., increasing the likelihood of pharma side-effects). This is serious - the patient could have significant liver damage or perhaps even die.

Note: If a patient take a prescription that states it should not be taken with grapefruit, they should speak to a physician about discontinuing that drug BEFORE beginning cannabis therapy, especially CBD-rich therapies).

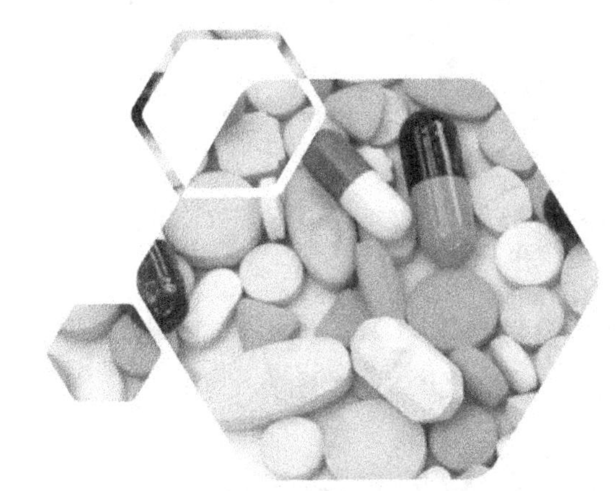

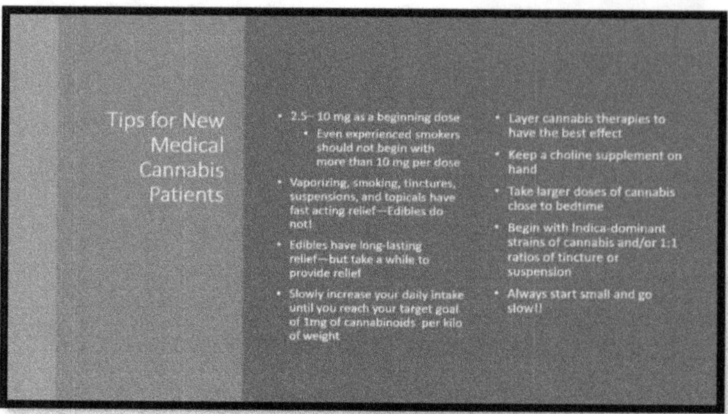

Tips for New Medical Cannabis Patients

•5 – 10 mg of "cannabinoids" as a beginning dose

Note: Even experienced smokers should not begin with more than 10 mg per dose

•Vaporizing, smoking, tinctures, suspensions, and topicals have fast acting relief—Edibles do not!

•Edibles have long-lasting relief—but take a while to provide relief, sometimes more than 2 hours.

•Slowly increase daily intake until the patient reaches the target goal of 1 mg of cannabinoids per kilo of weight

•Layer cannabis therapies to have the best effect

•Keep a choline supplement on hand

•Take larger doses of cannabis close to bedtime

•Begin with Indica-dominant strains of cannabis and/or 1:1 ratio of tincture or suspension

•**Always start small and go slow!!**

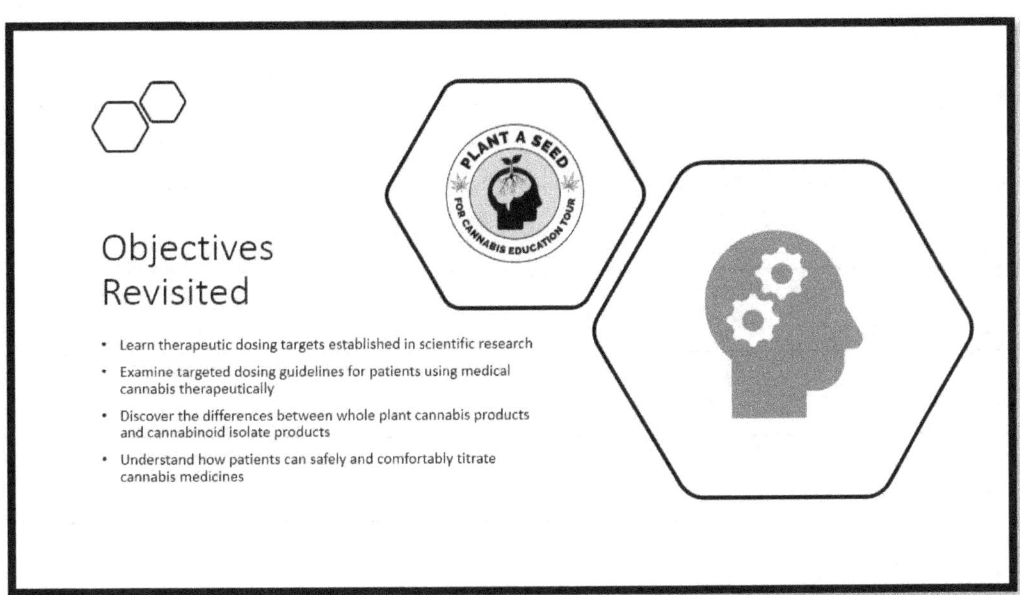

Objectives Revisited

PLANT A SEED
FOR CANNABIS EDUCATION TOUR

• Learn therapeutic dosing targets established in scientific research
• Examine targeted dosing guidelines for patients using medical cannabis therapeutically
• Discover the differences between whole plant cannabis products and cannabinoid isolate products
• Understand how patients can safely and comfortably titrate cannabis medicines

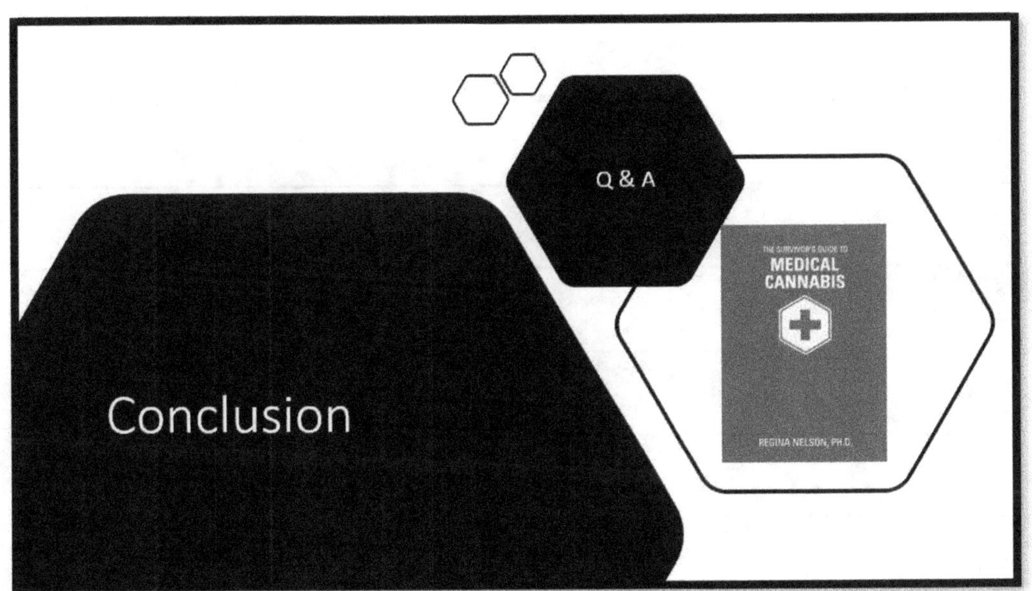

Q & A

THE SURVIVOR'S GUIDE TO
MEDICAL CANNABIS

REGINA NELSON, PH.D.

Conclusion

Notes

Notes

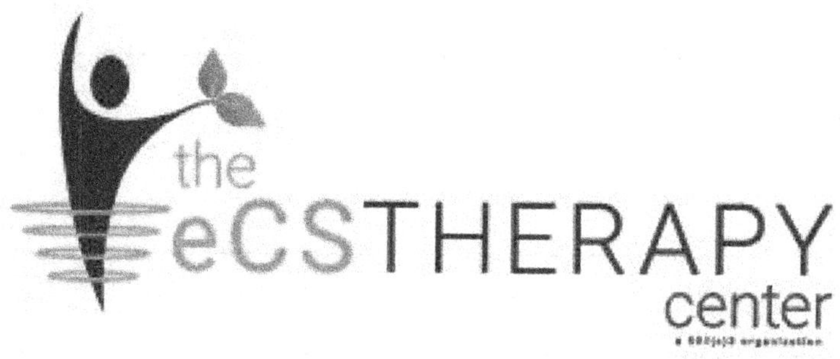

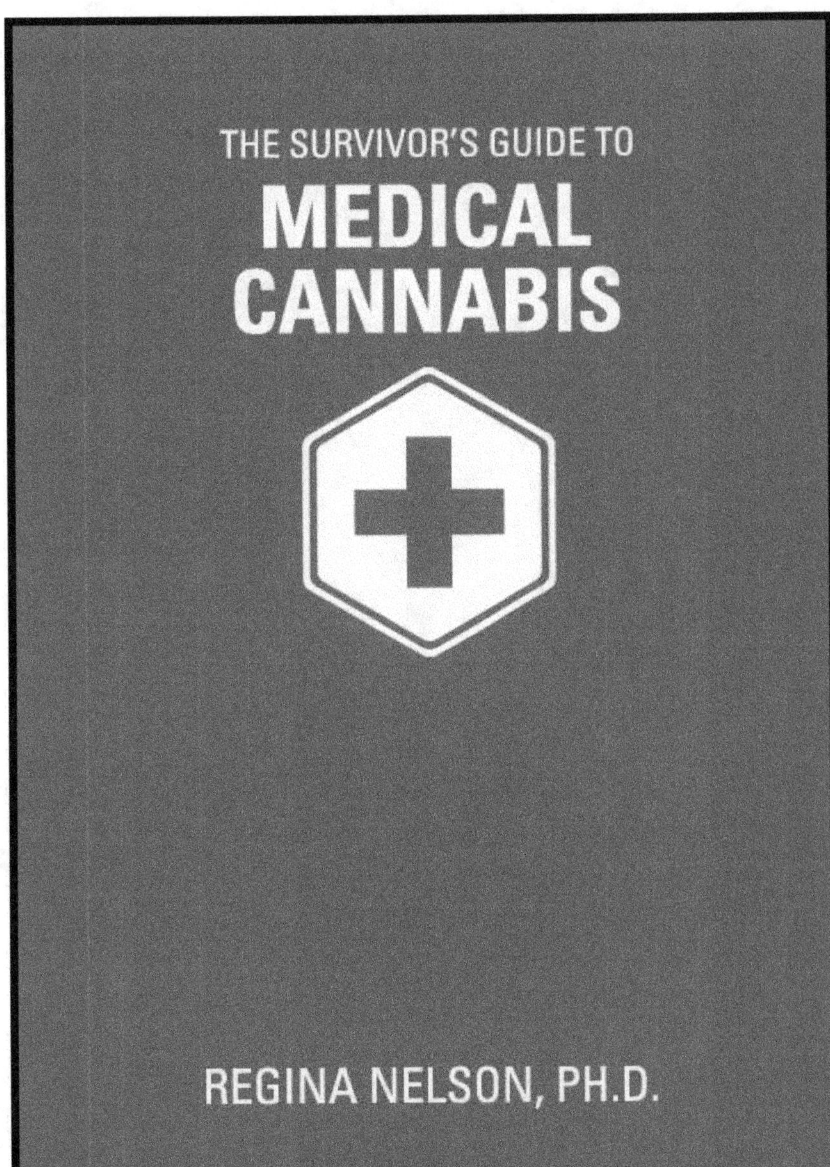

Available at
www.myecstherapy.org

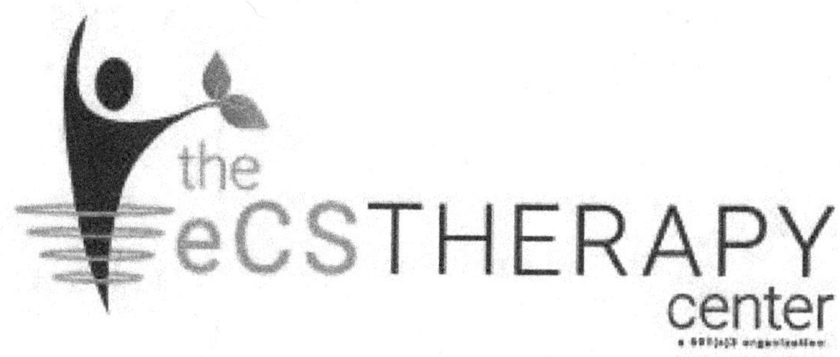

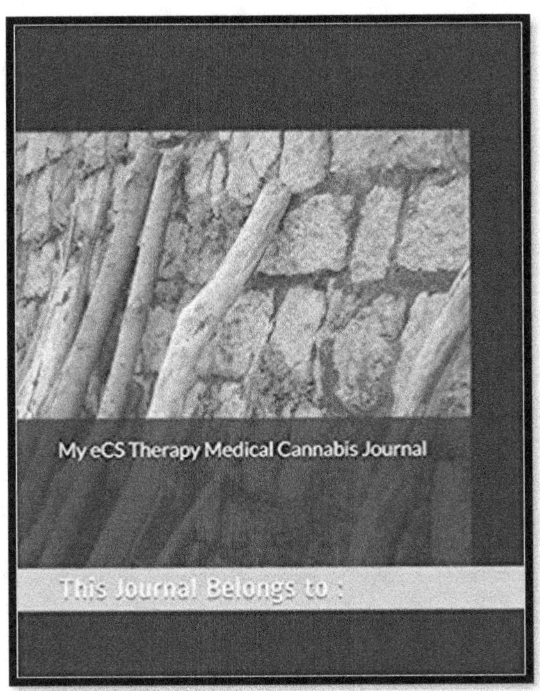

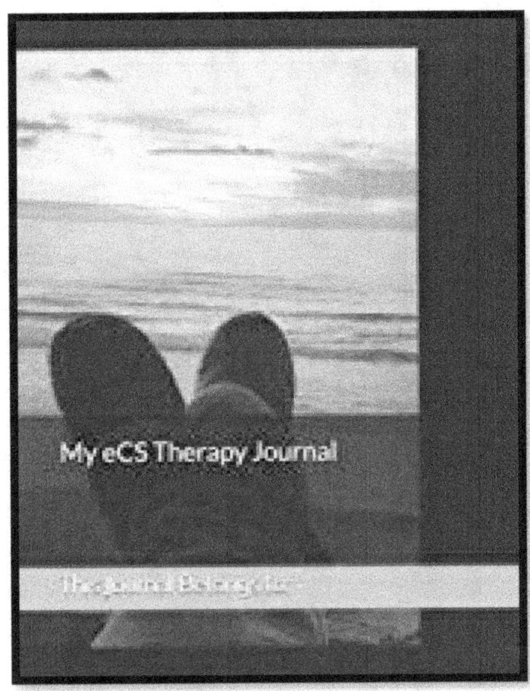

An EASY way to Journal
Get YOURS Today on Amazon
Or at www.MyECSTherapy>org

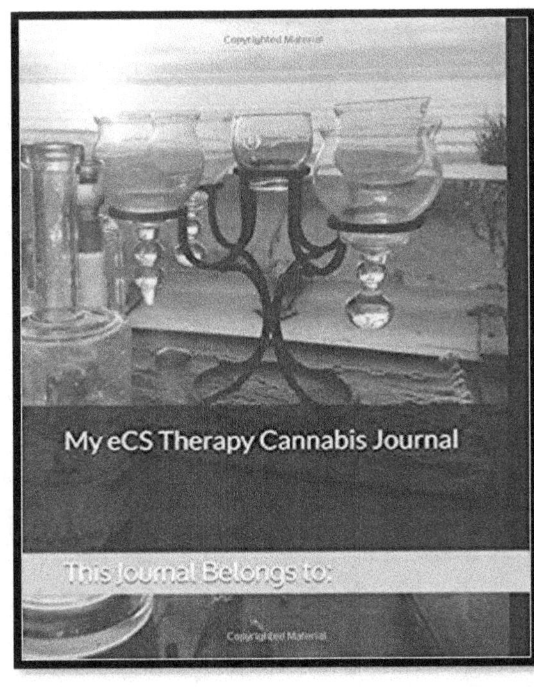

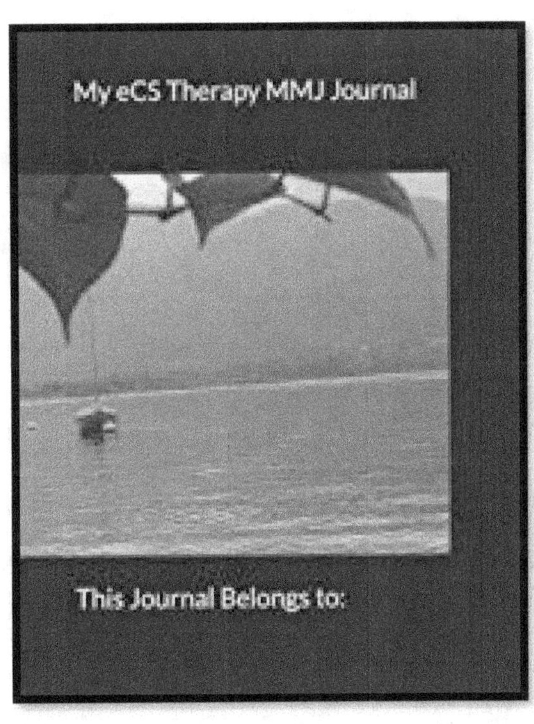

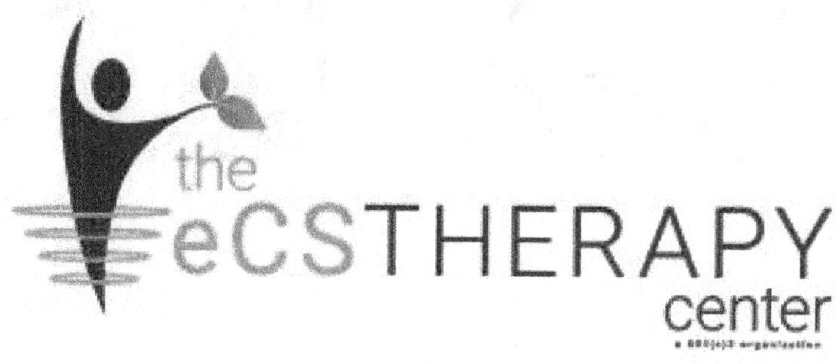

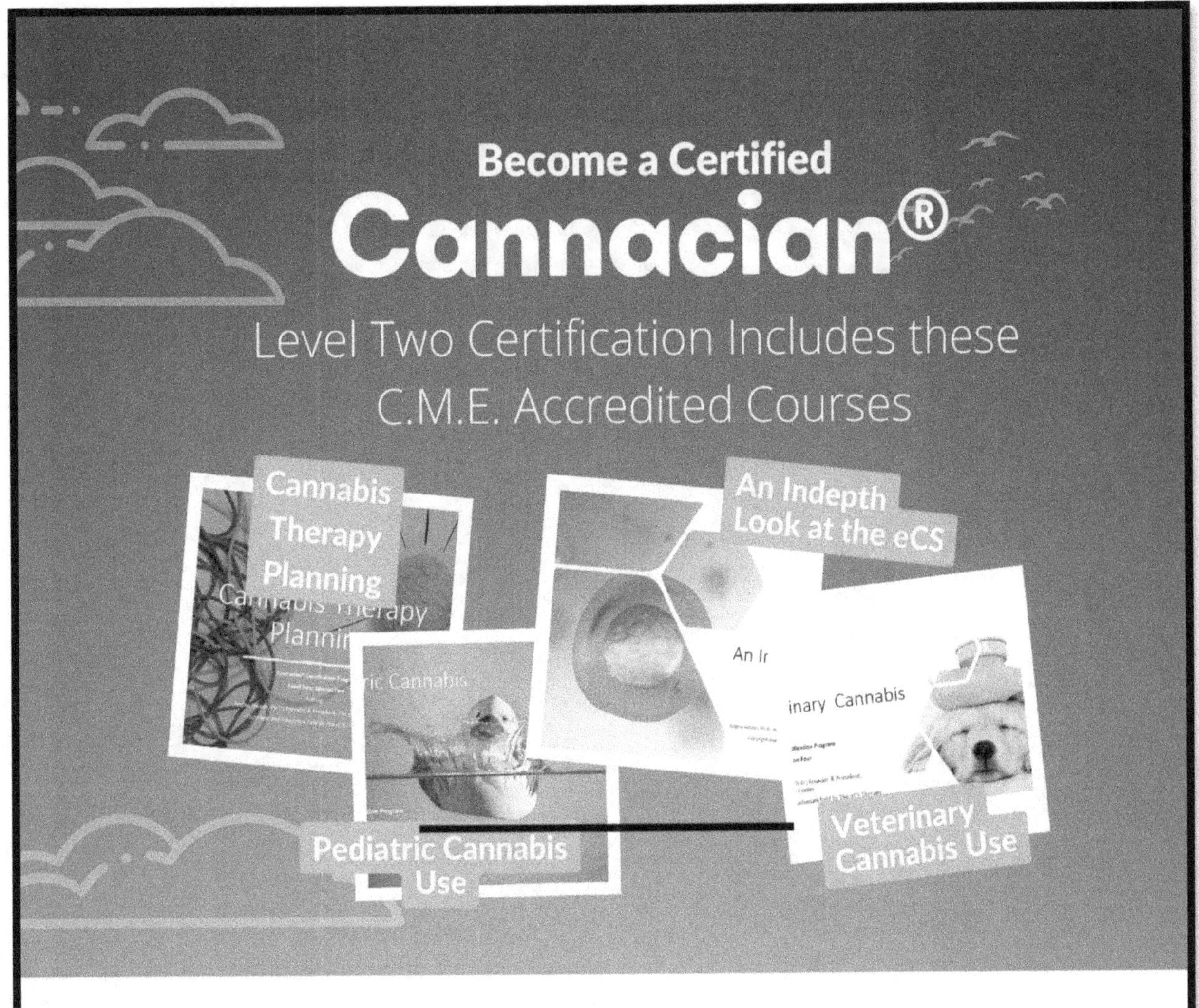

Take an Educated Step-Up!

www.myecstherapy.org

Bundle for Savings!

$349

All Three Cannacian Levels

Special Offer

Group Discounts

Up to 50%

price off/person

☑ 12 C.M.E. /C.E. Units Accredited A.A.F.P., A.V.A., and more

☑ Online via Teachable

☑ More than 12,000 Certified Cannacians World-wide

More info   Regina@myecstherapy.org

https://ecstherapycenter.teachable.com

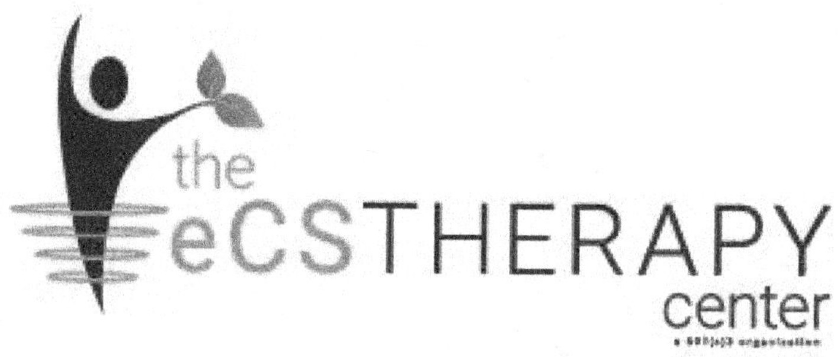

If you can't attend an event, join online!

https://ecstherapycenter.teachable.com

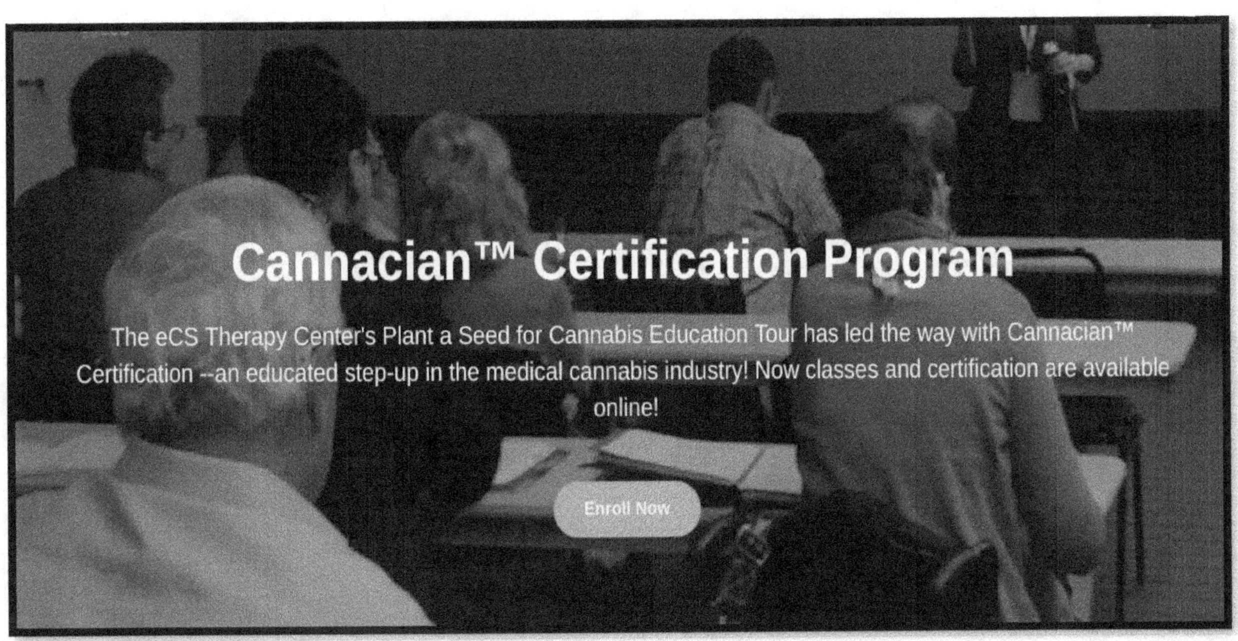

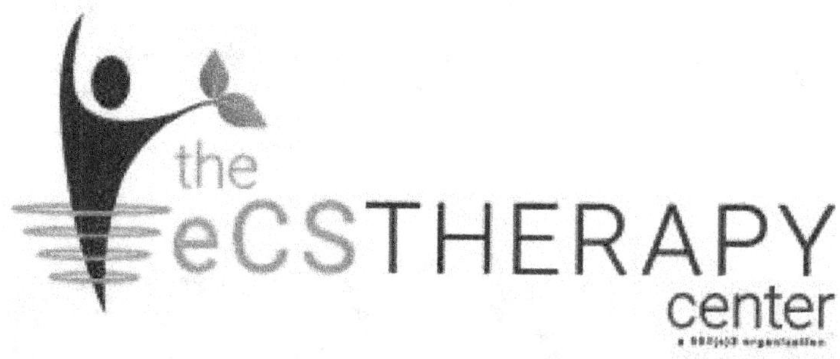

www.myecstherapy.org
Who is a
Cannacian®?
A COACH OR COUNSELOR
EDUCATED AND
KNOWLEDGEABLE ABOUT THE
USE OF CANNABIS AS
MEDICINE.
Cannacian® Certification offered by The eCS Therapy Center and from licensed
Cannacian® Trainers worldwide.

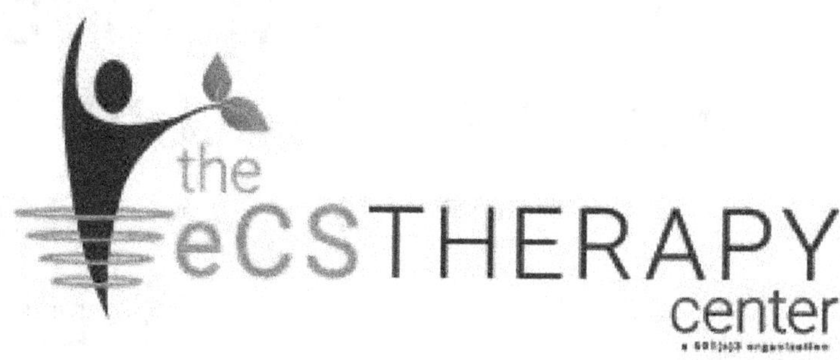
the
eCSTHERAPY
center
a 501(c)3 organization

Who is a Cannacian® Trainer?

Pronounced: /'kan-ni-SHən/

A Certified Cannacian® Trainer educates and certifies others using the Cannacian® program.

For more information visit:

www.myecstherapy.org

Regina@myecstherapy.org

A Cannacian® is a coach or counselor educated and knowledgeable about the use of cannabis as medicine.

**For certification visit:
https://ecstherapycenter
.teachable.com**

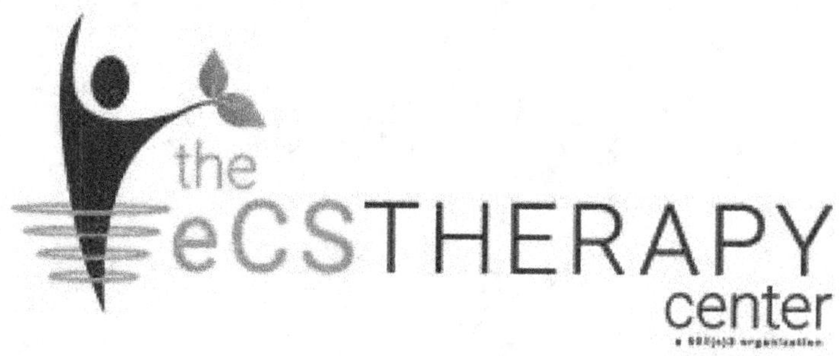

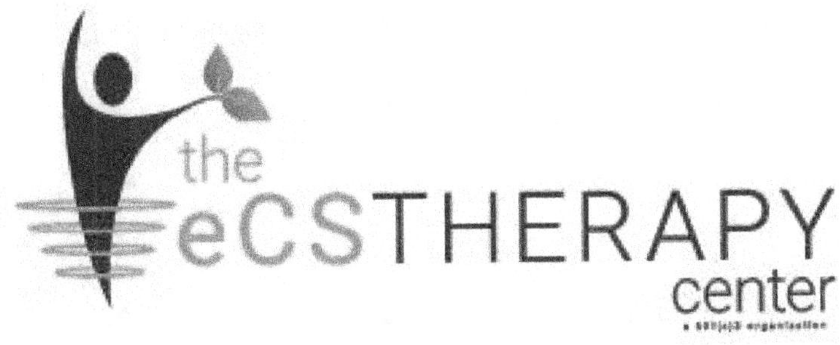